Yoga *and* Breast Cancer

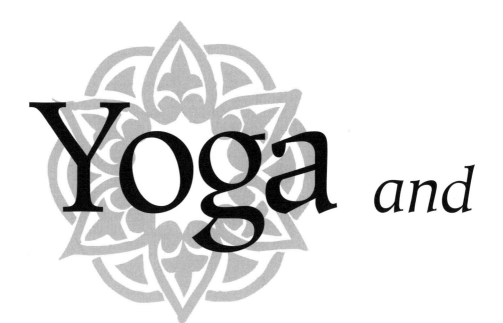

Yoga *and*

Breast Cancer

A Journey to Health and Healing

INGRID KOLLAK, RN, PhD

ISABELL UTZ-BILLING, MD

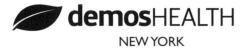

demosHEALTH

NEW YORK

Acquisitions Editor: Noreen Henson
Cover Design: Carlos Maldonado
Compositor: Absolute Service, Inc.
Printer: Bang Printing

Visit our Web site at www.demosmedpub.com

Library of Congress Cataloging-in-Publication Data

Kollak, Ingrid.
  Yoga and breast cancer : a journey to health and healing / Ingrid Kollak, Isabell Utz-Billing.
       p. cm.
  Includes bibliographical references and index.
   ISBN 978-1-932603-91-0 (alk. paper)
  1. Breast—Cancer—Patients—Rehabilitation. 2. Yoga—Therapeutic use. I. Utz-Billing, Isabell. II. Title.
   RC280.B8K65 2011
   616.99'44906—dc22
                                        2010030245

Special discounts on bulk quantities of Demos Health books are available to corporations, professional associations, pharmaceutical companies, healthcare organizations, and other qualifying groups. For details, please contact:

Special Sales Department
Demos Medical Publishing
11 W. 42nd Street
New York, NY 10036
Phone: 800–532–8663 or 212–683–0072
Fax: 212–941–7842
E-mail: rsantana@demosmedpub.com

Printed in the United States of America by Bang Printing.
10 11 12 13   5 4 3 2 1

*This book is dedicated to the women with
breast cancer who practiced yoga with us. They
shared their problems and concerns with us, as well as
their improvements and renewed confidence.
We could not have written this book
without them.*

Contents

PART II

YOGA FOR WOMEN WITH BREAST CANCER

PART III

YOGA POSTURES FOR MOMENTS IN BETWEEN

PART IV

CONCENTRATION AND MEDITATION

PART V

USEFUL INFORMATION

Foreword

Yoga has been practiced for 2,500 years, and it follows that it has been taught for very nearly that long. Tradition has it that in ancient times, yogis would attach themselves to great houses, serving as teachers, advisors, and healers. In those times yogis were known for their great knowledge as much as for the sweet reasonableness that seems to come unerringly to those that adhere to yogic practice. There is a certain calm that comes with the territory.

In those days, and indeed until quite recently, yoga was taught one-to-one. The pupil's undivided attention was fully reciprocated by the teacher. Focus, attentiveness, kindness with firmness, and many of the interpersonal virtues in yoga's Ten Commandments, the *Yamas* and *Niyamas*, were taught by precept and example in these two-person sessions. The parties got to know each other, and relationships naturally formed. Those wanting to become good yoga students did so through emulation as much as by resolving to follow yoga's principles. This may be why, after thousands of years of variegated practices and purposes, yoga has remained an astonishingly unitary thing.

But today, we have universities that specialize in teaching; psychiatrists, orators and analysts to advise us; and an entire medical and pharmaceutical industry to help us heal. Further, urban economics more or less requires that yoga be taught in groups. Yet yoga appears to be flourishing like never before.

Yoga must offer us something we need—something different from the learning, the advising, and even from the healing we are receiving from various pairs of expert hands.

In general terms, that something might be refuge: a hiatus in formal learning, a quieting of even the best advice, and a holiday from the disciplined healing on which one's very life may depend. Yoga appears to succeed in quieting the din, easing the restlessness, and softening the glare. Yoga offers an island of calm, a safe place of respite from any educational, commercial, or clinical efforts that take our time and attention. Like a "minimum daily requirement," it becomes obvious in its absence.

Ingrid Kollak, PhD, and Isabell Utz-Billing, MD, have created an anatomically knowledgeable and therapeutically focused volume that both teaches and exemplifies these principles. Like a barely perceptibly rising inclined plane, the book very gently lifts the breast cancer and post-breast cancer patient toward a realistic sense of well-being and inevitable joy with the improved health that accompanies it. This creates an ever-larger wedge between the "Cancer Patient" mentality and the "New Life" that the rigors of surgery and/or therapy have won for the yoga practitioner.

Ludwig Wittgenstein ended his first book with *"Wovon man nicht sprechen kann, darüber muß man schweigen,"* meaning "whereof we cannot speak, thereof must we be silent." The authors have almost self-consciously kept all the spiritual talk that abounds in the yoga world out of this volume. But their elegant pictures, simple contraindications, and thoughtful directions bear witness to the unassuming confidence and serenity with which the book was written, and that may be quite contagious.

Loren Fishman, MD

Acknowledgments

"You only need a casual outfit and a little bit of time," we told women in our flyer. Over a hundred women responded, saying they would take part in a study on yoga and its effects after breast cancer surgery. The study lasted from April 2008 through August 2009. The women involved met twice weekly to practice yoga as a group and were surveyed and interviewed before and after yoga practice regarding breast cancer, quality of life, and proper functioning of arms, shoulders, and neck. We thank those women. This book has grown out of that study, which combined our professional practice in yoga, our knowledge of medicine, and our intensive research.

We are thankful to Edel and Virginia who illustrate most of the postures and to our patients for their modeling and personal statements. We are grateful to our colleagues who collaborated with us during the study. We thank Marcel who spent long photo sessions with us and who visited us at the clinic. Our thanks go to Noreen Henson, our editor, who believed in the need for and interest in this book. Finally, special thanks to Anne Huntington and Amanda Cushman who reviewed the manuscript to make sure the book was enjoyable to read.

Yoga *and* Breast Cancer

PART
I

HOW TO USE THIS BOOK

The Importance of Yoga for Women with Breast Cancer

Yoga, with its different styles, intensities, and meditative methods, can be practiced by anyone. It is just a matter of finding the right style for your individual condition. This book details diverse versions of classical yoga asanas most suitable for women with breast cancer—even shortly after surgery. Yoga will help you become more aware of your body and mind, as well as your physical and mental well-being. You will learn to detect bad body positions and align your joints, to identify when you are stressed and alternate between tension and relaxation,

and to synchronize your breathing and harmonize your movements. Regular yoga practice—on your own or in a group—will help you feel better as you deal with the diagnosis and treatment of breast cancer.

Through text and photos, *Yoga and Breast Cancer* shows how yoga exercises enhance the quality of life for women diagnosed with breast cancer, wherever they might be in the stages of diagnosis, treatment, or recovery. This book offers support for women during the critical phases of their disease, as well as during times of rehabilitation and prevention.

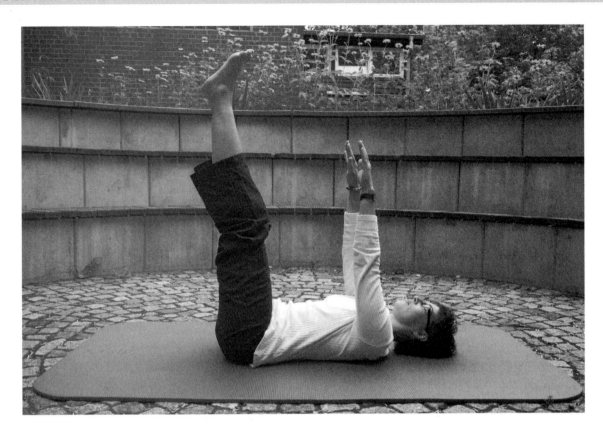

Yoga is a rich and elaborate approach to health and well-being—yoga is joy (yoga is bhoga). The foundation of yoga, the conscious coordination of breathing and movement, helps you enhance your flexibility and strength, reduce stress and anxiety, and teaches you to be self-reliant. The certainty of being able to rely on your own abilities and resources grows along with the experience needed to successfully master all kinds of challenges.

"I did yoga before—once in a while. This time yoga became vital to me. For the whole year my body was the theme of my yoga class: to regain my body, to think positively about my body, and to develop a new feeling for my body."

Our study showed that yoga has a positive influence on the mobility, flexibility, strength, and overall physical fitness of women undergoing treatment for breast cancer. And we are not the only researchers to draw this conclusion—our evidence corresponds with other published findings, such as those detailed in chapter 3. Women using yoga as part of a cancer recovery program will find that the exercises safely complement medical treatments and improve mental well-being by enhancing concentration and relaxation abilities. These skills, in turn, help them overcome anxiety and increase the body's healing ability. Finally, yoga helps women understand their breast cancer therapies and allows them to discover which exercises help overcome specific types of pain.

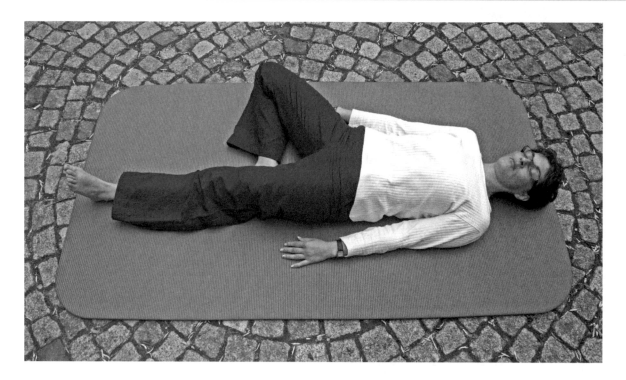

During our study, we focused on discovering which modifications of classical yoga exercises work best for women with breast cancer, particularly as they recover from surgery. Special care must be taken, but the benefits remain the same. First, through the practice of a variety of poses and movements, called asanas, yoga reduces physical pain by relaxing and stretching muscles and building strength and mobility. Second, yoga trains you to be aware of yourself, which helps you relax and helps reduce stress. The characteristic combination of movements and breathing rhythms makes the workout easier, calms the mind, and increases focus.

"During a time when you feel all kinds of loss, it's great to gain something. With yoga I became more flexible than I had been before my surgery."

Yoga is especially good for women with breast cancer because it is easy to perform soon after surgery, and its gentle movements allow you to be at ease with your new body.

"Even before I looked at my new breast, I put my drainage bottle into a little blue bag and went to the yoga class. That was pure comfort for me."

As you will see, each exercise in this book is accompanied by detailed information regarding proper alignment and breathing, which are necessary to prevent injury, but which also help you achieve relaxation and mobility in everyday life. The conscious coordination of breathing and movement used in yoga counteracts lasting tension and helps you gain flexibility, while the attention you pay to each movement allows you to feel the effects of an exercise as your brain registers sensations and identifies their locations. The awareness you gain of your body through yoga will allow you to recognize when your shoulders are tense, and you will also gain the ability to relieve that tension by relaxing and exhaling. With practice, you'll find that simple yoga exercises can be as effective as receiving a good massage. To find out which exercises benefit you the most, ask yourself: What does the asana do to your body and your mind? How does it affect the way you think? Does it feel good?

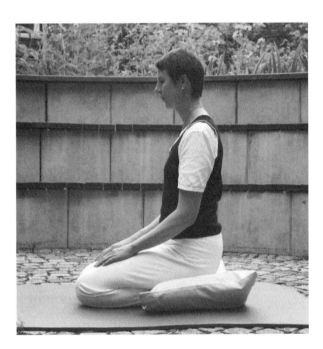

Yoga is special in that it addresses the physical *and* emotional afflictions experienced by women affected by breast cancer. Flowing movements enhance the mobility of your arms, relieve backaches or tight muscles; they keep you focused and help counteract recurring, troubling thoughts that create fear or sadness. When practicing yoga, you will feel the strength of the connection between body and mind.

"Yoga starts by affecting you physically. You begin by opening your arms and taking a deep breath. Slowly, you relax and begin to open yourself. I felt like a closed shell, and yoga offered me the chance to open myself. It is an offer. One is not forced to accept this offer. This is the core for me: Yoga offers a chance to open oneself."

As you continue to practice yoga, you become increasingly aware of your body, your mind, and your well-being. You learn to detect poor body alignment as well as burdening thoughts, and by navigating through mental and physical obstacles, you learn more about your personal resources. A better understanding of your body is a step toward a better understanding of your thoughts and feelings, and of your own inner strength.

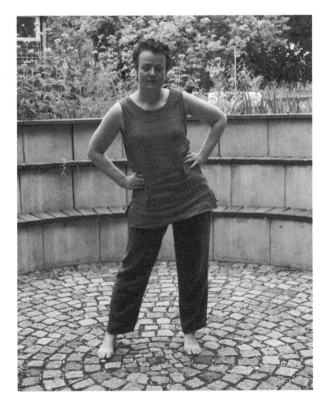

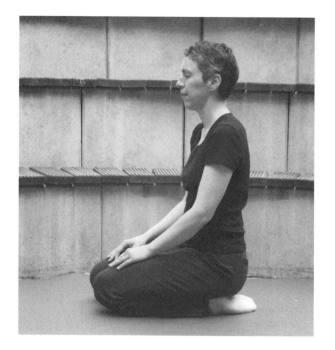

sensations, and emotions—is vital in learning to adjust how you feel. Breast cancer therapy can be devastating, and yoga exercises offer you the chance to do things differently and replace your usual thoughts and worries with a sense of joy. Changes in thinking patterns that start during practice spill over into everyday life, giving you a fresh outlook.

"In the midst of all the frightening information there came a person who offered something positive: a yoga class. And because I already knew yoga, I was sure it would be the right thing to do. I thought: What a great idea!"

Practicing yoga offers you a number of paths to understanding your inner strength. Through increased attention to your own thoughts, the sensations in your body, and the emotions that you feel as you end a position, you will come to understand yourself. Sharpening the degree to which you can focus your awareness to each of these aspects—thoughts,

We wrote this book for women with breast cancer who are interested in practicing yoga as a special way to actively overcome their disease and to reunite with their body. Using the yoga exercises presented here, you will learn to mitigate difficulties after surgery and during therapy, to improve awareness of your body, thoughts, and feelings, and to lead a healthier life.

2

Our Study

When we started our study about the effects of yoga on breast cancer patients, we knew that regular yoga practice can improve the physical and psychological well-being of women, but were unsure of how good it would be for women with breast cancer.

We wanted to prove that yoga could help women with breast cancer regain their physical capacities more quickly, as well as rediscover their love for themselves. We all know that breast cancer treatments are very difficult for women to endure, but some earlier studies had suggested that yoga could not only ease a woman's discomfort but also improve her overall well-being. We wanted to corroborate this.

Yoga classes met twice a week. A yoga instructor who had been diagnosed with breast cancer herself fifteen years ago led the group alternately with Dr. Ingrid Kollak. We concentrated on strengthening and relaxing exercises, ensuring that each participant found her own optimal degree of intensity for each exercise.

To find out the specific effects of yoga on breast cancer patients, we asked our volunteers to complete standardized questionnaires about their physical and mental well-being, their quality of life, and their social support systems at the beginning of the course and after its completion. Furthermore, we interviewed women about their feelings and state-of-mind. Patients were randomly placed into two groups. The first group started practicing yoga as early as two to three days after their first operation. These patients even came to their first class with drainage tubes. The second group started five to six weeks later.

And the result—yoga really helps patients with breast cancer! It trains concentration and attentiveness. Participants can find inner peace and strength. They learn to better understand their own needs. In this way, they build their strength in order to conquer their illness, but also to find their own personal way through the many tips and recommendations they receive.

All women with breast cancer should consider using the time following their operation and any necessary further treatment to improve their physical and psychological well-being through regular yoga practice. With the help of yoga, you can regain mobility and strength more rapidly. Breathing exercises are helpful with nausea. Yoga practice can also help you to correct compensatory postures that are unconsciously established following an operation.

The study's participants loved our lessons, and everyone chose to continue their yoga practice after completion of the study—the best outcome we could have hoped for.

3

Current Studies on Breast Cancer and Yoga

Yoga has become a popular subject of medical inquiry and is now being studied by many clinicians. Known for its therapeutic benefits, yoga is now offered as a complementary therapy at many major treatment centers, and is often practiced independently by patients who hear how effective it is.

For women with breast cancer, yoga has been shown to reduce mood disturbance, anxiety, depression, anger, stress, and confusion, and to improve sleep quality, cancer related distress, and cancer related symptoms.[1,3–5,21] Women participating in yoga programs during treatment reported improvements in their quality of life—for example, there was a significant reduction in nausea, vomiting, and fatigue during chemotherapy.[8,11,12,18,19]

Other studies have examined the impact of yoga on a sampling of patients with metastatic breast cancer. The findings suggest that, along with improvement in pain control and relaxation, yoga significantly boosted energy and helped the women accept their condition.[7]

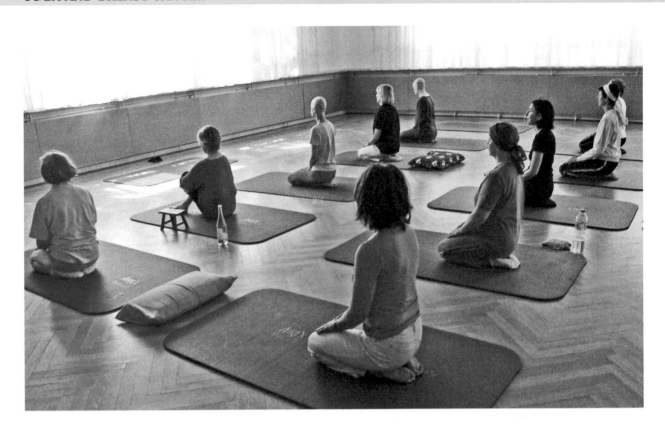

As you begin your practice, you will find that yoga impacts your health in a variety of ways. For example, many women with breast cancer who receive hormonal treatments suffer from menopausal symptoms. A comprehensive yoga program has been shown to control symptoms such as hot flashes, sleep disturbance, and fatigue, and symptoms related to changes in mood and energy levels. Studies have demonstrated that yoga produces a relaxation response by integrating a set of changes, including increased breath volume and decreased heart rate.[22] Yoga also produces invigorating effects on mental and physical energy, similar to the effects of aerobic exercise, and may thereby improve sleep and reduce fatigue.[7,9]

Those with concerns more mental than physical will also find help through yoga.

Struggling to control your sensations, thoughts, or emotions is often counterproductive, and research shows that the effort to control such things produces heightened psychological distress and increased sympathetic activation.[15] From its origins, yoga emphasizes acceptance of one's moment-to-moment experiences, whatever they may be.[7] By learning this skill, you will find yourself more relaxed in your day-to-day life.

Finally, yoga, as a gentler physical activity, may promote regular participation in exercise. For those who suffer from chronic conditions, this is particularly important, since it can be difficult for them to engage in active lifestyles.[2,16] As you recover from surgery or cope with therapy, yoga offers a fulfilling yet manageable way to stay healthy.

4

How to Use This Book

Yoga and Breast Cancer was written especially for women with breast cancer who are undergoing therapy, recovering from their illness, or interested in further prevention. Relatives and friends of these women might also be interested in the advice given in these pages. With a focus on the practical uses of yoga, we show you how to use yoga to manage stress and relieve pain, and how to find a proper level of self-care that both reduces your vulnerability and enhances your resistance. The in-depth exploration of the effects of yoga will help you find the style most suited to your body and mind, guiding you toward the start of your own yoga program. Through the study and practice of the various yoga postures presented here, you will grow stronger both physically and mentally, and be on your way to a healthier life.

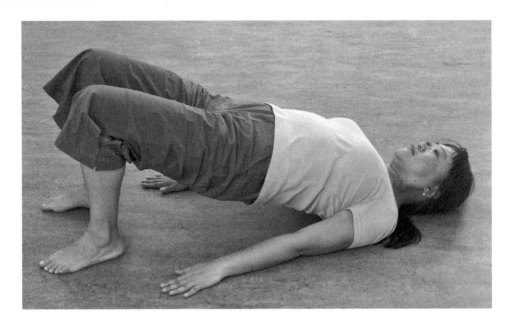

Women with breast cancer are not the only ones who can benefit from understanding the relationship between yoga and recovery. We also hope to attract the attention of professionals who work with breast cancer patients, including physicians, nurses, physical therapists, psychotherapists, and counselors of self-help groups. Yoga teachers interested in offering classes for women after breast cancer surgery will find helpful suggestions in these pages.

> *"It is wonderful that there are no obligations during the yoga class. As a patient, one is burdened with obligations—obligations that are quite unpleasant."*

The yoga postures and their variations, as shown in this book, were developed with the assistance of over one hundred women over a period of eighteen months. The program we established during our study is systematic from head to toe, meaning you can follow the comprehensive guide—which includes step-by-step explanations, descriptions of corresponding breathing techniques, and photographs of each exercise—as you develop your own exercising rhythm. In addition, when you perform yoga exercises throughout the day accompanied by the correct synchronized breathing technique, you will feel better immediately and will increase your concentration and energy. The exercises presented in part III, "Yoga Postures for Moments in Between," are especially good for this.

The variety of yoga postures presented here will allow you to enjoy your yoga practice no matter your preferences, abilities, or location. And because you feel the effects of each exercise immediately, you can adjust postures as needed to remain comfortable. Finally, if you begin yoga and would like to practice in a group, you can easily find yoga classes and teachers in your area.

"There is no higher, faster, better. There is no comparison with others. It is just you and yoga."

Though these asanas encompass a large variety of movements, they are all easily doable in their *modified* versions. The modifications are intended to meet your needs following surgery or as a beginner. We also show *variations*, for example, using a chair or a cushion, or bending one arm, that help during periods of therapy when you are less flexible. In our study, women happily continued the class with the help of props even when they felt groggy or weak. To avoid strain or injury, continue with the modified versions until you are aware of the effects these asanas have on your body and mind. Once you have practiced for a while, or if you practiced yoga previously and know what these variations and more difficult modes can do for you, you may consider doing the more challenging *reference* postures.

All the asanas in this book are carefully described and serve the needs of women who want to actively support their therapies and enhance their physical fitness as well as their mental well-being while dealing with breast cancer. If you would like to learn more, we have listed Web pages in the back of this book about the best-known hatha yoga traditions.

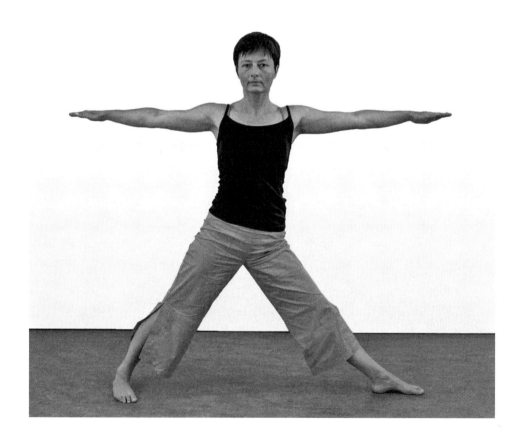

5

Practical Advice for Beginning Yoga Practice

There are no medical contraindications for the practice of the following yoga postures and exercises. Don't be afraid of injuring yourself by reopening the wound, for example, while performing the movements; your body will tell you which exercises you can do without hurting yourself. You can practice after an operation even if you still have a drainage tube (the flexible tube placed in the wound to drain blood and secretions from the wound, which will be removed a few days after the surgery). Start moving your arms as soon as possible after surgery to maintain and develop your strength and mobility. If you feel any pain, slow down, even if you are in a class. Do not feel pressed to complete an asana—just trust your own judgment. As you exercise, you will begin to recognize what each posture does to you, how it feels, and which ones feel good. With time, the practice of yoga will help you become accustomed to the changes in your body after surgery.

THE RIGHT TIME TO BEGIN YOGA

According to the approximately two-thousand-year-old Sanskrit yoga sutras, which form the foundation of all hatha yoga practice today, those who practice yoga attentively are able to practice it for years and enjoy it into old age. But when, and how, should you begin?

Yoga provides benefits only through practice, so we recommend you start with the modified yoga postures detailed in this book within a day or two after your surgery. The changes in your body, including increased flexibility and mobility following the initial post-surgery stiffness, will convince you of yoga's effectiveness. You may also be surprised by your ability to fight through not wanting to exercise.

When we asked the women in our group when to start yoga, most of them agreed it was better to start early:

"In my opinion, the earlier you start, the better. I started five weeks after my surgery. When I saw women practicing with a drainage tube in their wounds, I thought I should have started earlier. I could have avoided the feelings of stiffness and immobility that I had at first."

"For me it was good to start yoga immediately after the surgery. I knew I was in the need of something that would give me time to get used to my new body. In the yoga class I had time to get in touch with my body, my mind, my breath. It was a great help to me."

For others, it was not as important that they start immediately after surgery. Only you can decide what the right time, and reason, are for you. For example, some women in our group loved to do sports and quickly resumed their regular activities by doing gymnastics, riding their bikes, or taking walks. Their physical fitness came back easily, but they told us that they couldn't cope with the situation when therapy was over. Their need for yoga was mental and emotional.

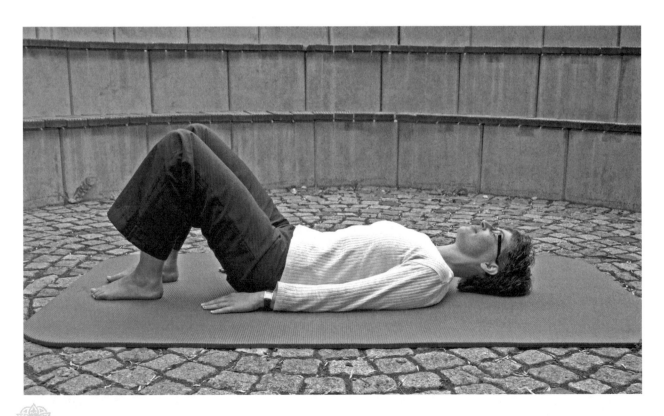

"In my case, my despair did not start the day after my surgery but about six weeks later. It was very severe. I wouldn't call it depression, but I was very distressed at that time. It was good that I started practicing yoga when I felt weak and my courage had left me."

DEVELOP YOUR INDIVIDUAL YOGA PRACTICE

Whenever you decide it's best for you to start, make it a habit from the beginning by keeping to your yoga time and maintaining your rhythm. Make yoga enjoyable by approaching it playfully. Yoga starts with the practice and understanding of the postures and counterpostures, but developing a conscious yoga practice is vital. The key to developing this conscious practice is to keep to a fixed rhythm. Always start the exercises from the same side of the body—the ancient hatha yoga pradipika manual recommends the left side—and repeat the exercises for the same length of time. For beginners, we recommend six complete inhalations and exhalations, the equivalent of six complete movements. Regular practice of the yoga postures will help you deepen your understanding of their significance and allow you to adapt the postures to your needs. Experienced yoga students know when they need a special stretch, an extra bend, or a certain resting posture.

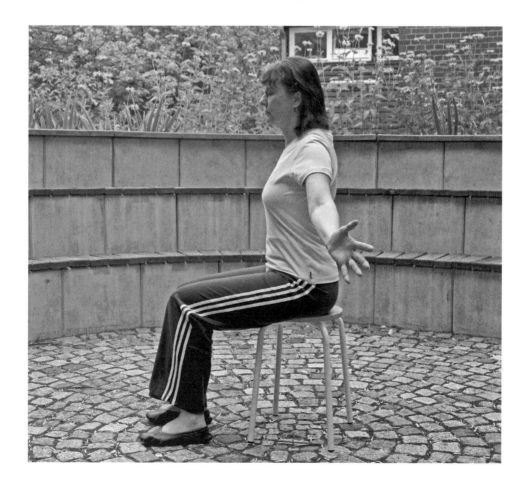

HOW TO PREPARE FOR YOGA

Wear comfortable clothes, such as sweatpants and t-shirts that feel good and sit well. Practice yoga with bare feet whenever you can.

Use a nonslip yoga mat or exercise on the floor, and use a blanket for all relaxing, breathing, and concentrating exercises. Roll up a blanket and use it as a bolster for your knees or as a support for your head if you prefer or need it.

Inhale and exhale through your nose. We marked the few exceptions to this rule.

Maintain your breathing rhythm while practicing yoga. As a beginner, try to complete six deep inhalations and exhalations, the equivalent of six complete movements.

Start exercising with your eyes open, closing them only at the end of an exercise, or after you worked on the first side, if it helps you feel the effects. After some practice, you might even prefer to exercise with your eyes closed.

Always start the exercises on the same side of the body.

If possible, practice at the same place and time. This makes it easier to watch your improvements and become aware of your current strengths and weaknesses.

You will always feel better once you get going.

KEEPING A PERSONAL JOURNAL

As you begin to practice yoga, you might like to find ways of incorporating postures and breathing techniques into your daily life. A personal journal gives you a place to write down your goals, determine options for achieving those goals, formulate a plan of action, and document your progress. Studying the journal can help you understand the reasons for successes and failures, and to build on them. Though learning yoga is virtually guaranteed to improve the quality of your life, your first attempts, as with any new activity, may be clumsy and slow. You may feel unsure of yourself and ready to give up. Have courage and continue. Do each exercise step by step as we show you in this book, and try keeping a personal journal.

If you decide you want to try using a personal journal, get a nice note pad or open a new file on your computer. Make two columns: one in which you note what you want to achieve and when, and the other in which you write down what you have done, including any comments, thoughts, and ideas. Make sure that your goals are specific; instead of writing "less pain" or "feel better," write "keep my spine stretched" or "do the lion when feeling sad." Your actions should be something that you want to do, that you realistically can do, and that bring you closer to a healthier life.

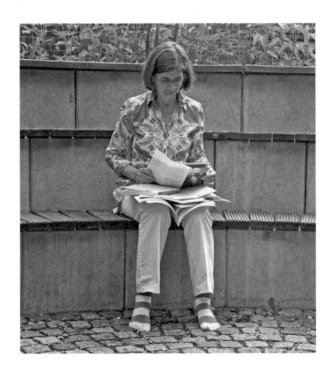

When coming up with an action plan, ask yourself: What do you want to achieve? Which asanas are you going to practice? How often and how much do you want to practice? At what time do you want to practice? With whom do you want to practice? When evaluating your actions, recognize any new skills, changes in energy, and alterations in your well-being. Don't forget to credit your successes and use them to bolster further progress. Note:

How often you practice.
The effects on your shoulders and arms.
Comparisons before and after the exercise.
Differences between your left and right arm.
Improvements to your flexibility.
Thoughts you have while practicing.
Progress and obstacles in your daily practice.

Confidence is vital for recovery, and learning yoga boosts confidence. You

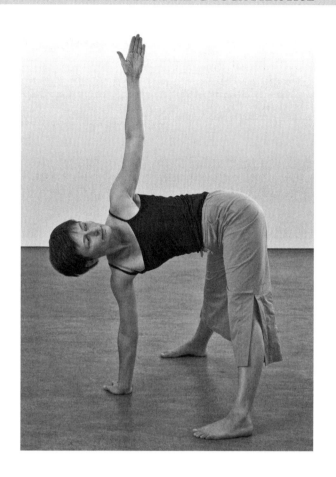

EXAMPLE OF AN ACTION PLAN	
Goals	**Results**
Ease the pain in the shoulders and left arm.	I repeated the Hero 1 posture six times and kept the posture through two complete breaths. My arms felt lighter after the exercise. Asked Noreen (neighbor in yoga class) about her experience with yoga after radiation. She thinks it has helped her. Talked about the "white light imagination."
Work on Hero 1 posture and practice it for six movements during my yoga class tomorrow.	
Exercise Hero 1 three times a day until Friday: After waking-up, before radiation, and before going to bed.	I feel as if I have gained length in my spine. Felt groggy after radiation but slept through the night after.
Stretch my spine when standing and waiting, and after entering the car.	
Ask my yoga neighbor about her experience with yoga and radiation.	
White light imagination?	

EXAMPLE OF AN ACTION PLAN	
Goals	**Results**
Ease the pain in the lower back. Compare the knee-to-chest posture on a mat during class and in bed after waking up.	I tried the knee-to-chest posture one week in the class (twice) and after waking up every morning! The warmth of the bed was a comfortable place to get started and stretch the whole spine. The results of the posture may have been better when practiced on the mat. I will continue trying it both ways.

master postures, solve problems, learn and get support from others, and help women in the same situation. As you continue practicing, you will feel more in control of your new situation. Before this assurance becomes apparent within you in daily life, you will observe it in your yoga practice. The more you focus on your breathing and movement, as well as on proper alignment, the more you learn to rely on yourself. This self-reliance, in turn, gives you the strength to master your illness.

The journal can also help you keep track of different ways you've tried to accomplish a certain goal.

A journal can also help you apply yoga to your daily life by helping you note new competencies, stay on track, and learn how to enhance your well-being. If you can gain more strength and flexibility and lower your stress level, you will gain energy and confidence. Don't expect too much, but make sure you note your progress and honor it.

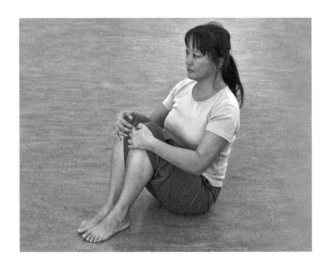

"We used to think in black and white. But what do we mean by healthy and what do we mean by sick? Are they opposing qualities? Is there only ever one of them present at a time? I prefer to ask what they have in common. One cannot exist without the other. I had to be sick to lead the healthy life I am leading today. After my first shock, I reconciled. I reduced my work and slowed down. I take myself more seriously now and I prefer my new life to my old one."

PART
II

YOGA FOR WOMEN WITH

BREAST CANCER

6

How to Begin: Basic Stances

Yoga can be done by anyone and should be a joy (bhoga). To get the most out of your practice, start by choosing the basic stances that work best for you and your body. Experiment with the recommended variations, and don't hesitate to use a prop if it helps you feel comfortable. In our study group, some women began their postures seated in a chair while others chose to kneel.

> *"I would have been disappointed if I had been asked to come into a kneeling posture while I was getting hormonal treatments and suffering from stiffness in my ankles. I loved the freedom to choose from a variety of yoga postures. And it impressed me that I was told to practice in accordance with my actual fitness."*

In this section, we present basic stances and their variations. Again, keep in mind your own level of fitness and choose the variation that feels right to you.

Purposes

The basic stances—done standing, sitting, kneeling, or lying on the floor—are essential to every yoga posture. When performed properly, they enhance your overall posture, deepen your breathing, and support your ability to focus.

Each posture in yoga begins with a proper basic stance. As you gain experience, you will find that by taking this stance you immediately become aware of how your body feels, of the depth and rhythm of your breathing, and of your thoughts, feelings, and mood. Returning to this stance between exercises, or after the first half of a posture, gives you the opportunity to assess how your body feels compared to before the exercise.

Finally, and perhaps most importantly, the basic stances are a fundamental part of your breathing, concentration, and meditation postures. The first yoga scholars used only a small number of seated postures for meditation, mastering the one that best enabled them to listen to their teacher and practice various techniques. Today, the basic postures serve a similar purpose in sharpening your focus on yourself and your practice.

Contraindications

There are no contraindications to the basic stances. However, they can be made easier in some ways. Some can be difficult on your knees, and if you find it uncomfortable to kneel on your heels, use a bolster (folded blanket) placed under either your knees or your feet as a prop. If you at first lack the flexibility to do seated postures on the floor, you can gradually improve your flexibility by sitting on a cushion while exercising. If you suffer from uncontrolled high blood pressure or from eye and ear conditions, rest your head on a cushion or folded blanket so that your head is raised above your heart level. Finally, rising suddenly from a calm stance can lead to a decrease in blood pressure and make you feel dizzy, so go slowly and inhale while rolling upward into a standing position or while gently moving into the next asana.

Alignments

In all the basic stances, the spinal column is stretched out from your pelvis to the crown of your head. Feel the stretch in your neck. In seated or standing postures, your chin is parallel to the ground, whereas in supine postures (lying on the back), your chin points toward your chest. Relax your shoulders and arms, as well as your face and tongue muscles, and breathe slowly in and out through your nose. More specific information is given for each basic stance described in the next few pages.

"It was good to start the yoga class lying on the back. It gave you a chance to adjust to the place and the ambiance. And it felt good to slowly move up, to be aware of the body during and after each yoga exercise."

LYING ON THE BACK

All supine postures start from this basic stance. Lie on your back with your body stretched out completely, arms by your sides.

Basic Stance

Lie on the floor.

Stretch your neck with your chin pointing toward your chest.

Stretch your back and legs; flex your feet so that your toes point toward the ceiling.

Stretch your arms out next to your body, palms facing down.

Let your face, lips, and tongue relax.

Breathe in and out deeply through your nose.

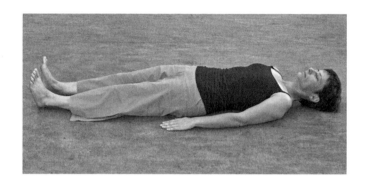

Variation with a Cushion

If you have uncontrolled high blood pressure or ear and eye conditions, place your head on a cushion or folded blanket.

Variation with Bent Knees

If you have difficulty stretching your legs or if the lower part of your back is not completely flat on the floor, bend your knees and place your feet flat on the floor, hip width apart.

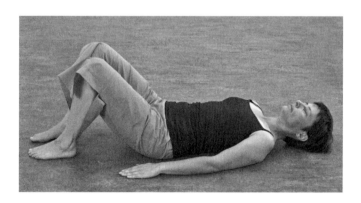

UPRIGHT SEATED POSTURES

Seated Posture on a Chair

If you have trouble sitting or kneeling on the floor (which can be the case if your joints are stiff during hormonal treatment), use this stance. Also try to assume this position occasionally during the day; for example, when you're seated at a table or riding in a car, because it will help stretch your spine and open your chest.

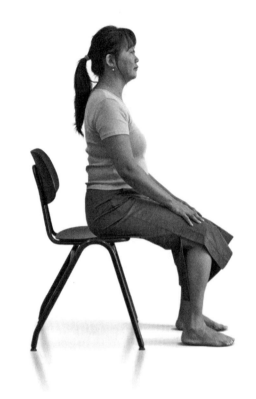

Sit down on a chair and distribute your weight evenly on both sit bones (buttocks).

Position your feet hip width apart. The weight of your legs should be evenly distributed on your feet. The outer edges of your feet are parallel to one another.

Position your knee joints directly above your ankles.

Pull your pelvis upright, stretch your spinal column, and extend the crown of your head upward.

Raise your sternum and lay your hands loosely on your thighs.

Align your chin parallel to the floor, and relax your face, lips, and tongue.

Breathe in and out deeply through your nose.

Upright Seated Posture on the Floor

It takes a bit of practice to sit on the floor with your legs stretched out in front of you, but this posture is useful to start with because it allows you to adjust your pelvis and vertebrae. Bending forward or backward from this position strengthens your back and belly muscles, which are especially important during treatment periods when you might not have enough strength in your arms to pull yourself up.

Sit on the floor and distribute your weight evenly on both sit bones.

Position your feet hip width apart.

Flex your feet and pull your toes in the direction of your belly.

Pull your pelvis upright, stretch your spinal column, and extend the crown of your head upward.

Raise your sternum and lay your hands loosely on your thighs.

Align your chin parallel to the ground, and relax your face, lips, and tongue.

Breathe in and out deeply through your nose.

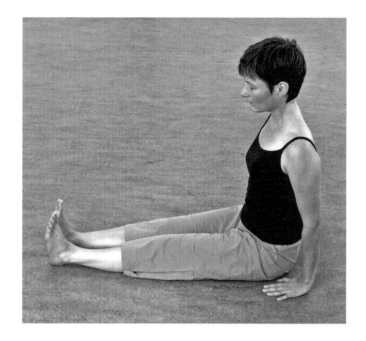

Variations with Hands on the Floor or with a Bolster

If your back muscles are too weak to maintain the upright posture, use one of these variations to avoid getting into a humpbacked position. Either place both hands on the floor on either side of your pelvis, or place a blanket or bolster under your sit bones.

Upright Seated Posture with Crossed Legs

Because it is more important to stretch your back than your knees, bend your knees in the beginning if it feels more comfortable.

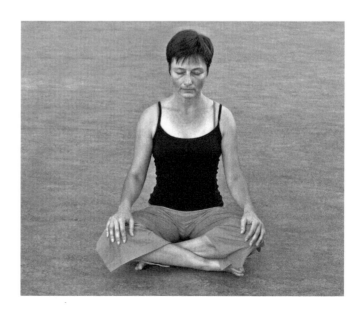

KNEELING POSTURES

The kneeling postures, which are particularly beneficial for some breathing techniques, can be difficult at first, so you may find it easier to use a stool or a bolster.

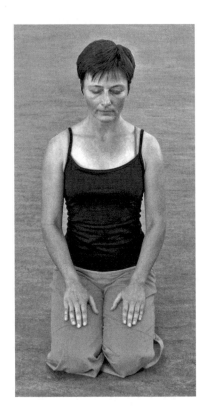

Sit on the floor with your sit bones resting on your heels. Your feet are stretched, your toes are pointed and facing inward, and the tops of your feet are flat on the floor.

Pull your pelvis into an upright position, tighten your pelvic muscles, and relax your belly.

Straighten your spinal column, and raise your sternum.

Relax your shoulders and arms, and rest your hands on your thighs.

Align your chin parallel to the floor, and relax your face, lips, and tongue.

Breathe in and out deeply through your nose.

Variation with a Cushion

If the kneeling posture is uncomfortable for either your knees or your ankles, use a cushion or folded blanket to relieve pressure. Because there are a couple of ways to use a bolster in this position, try both to determine which works best for you. First, try placing the cushion between your upper and lower legs, and see how that feels.

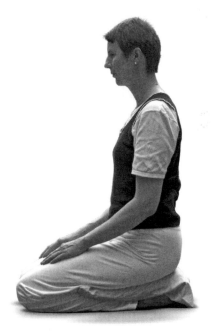

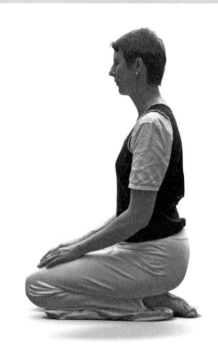

Then, try placing the cushion under your knees and ankles and compare. By experimenting, you can determine which placement works best for you.

Variation with a Stool

If you find it difficult to sit on your heels, (if, for example, your leg muscles are too tight and there is too much space between your sit bones and your heels) use a prop, preferably a small stool. If you don't have a stool, use a bolster.

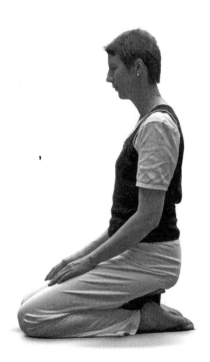

STANDING POSTURE

While many yoga postures start from the standing basic stance, the standing posture can also be an asana in itself: the mountain posture. Though it looks quite ordinary, the mountain posture is one of the most beneficial postures when done properly and performed often throughout the day. The burden of dealing with breast cancer and therapy can make you feel small and affect your posture by causing you to hunch over. By performing the mountain posture, you will raise yourself up and stand tall, helping yourself calm down, lower your shoulders, and relax your face. You can quickly feel the influence of the posture in both body and mind.

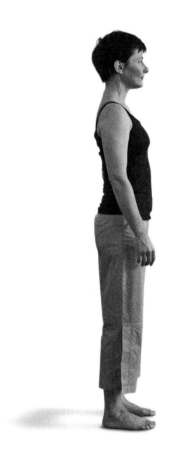

Place your feet hip width apart, and distribute the weight of your body evenly on your feet. If you feel more weight on the inner side of your feet (a tendency toward standing knock-kneed), make sure that you correct your weight distribution toward the outer edges of your feet (and vice versa).

Extend your knees without hyperextending (locking) them.

Rotate your thighs outward, keeping your feet in place; feel your pelvis lifting up.

Support the position of your pelvis by tightening your pelvic muscles.

Stretch your vertebrae between your tailbone and the crown of your head.

Relax your belly.

Raise your sternum, and let your shoulders and arms hang down loosely.

Align your chin parallel to the floor, and relax your face, lips, and tongue.

Breathe in and out deeply through your nose.

QUICK LOOK

Chapter 6 HOW TO BEGIN: BASIC STANCES	
Lying on the Back	All supine postures start from this basic stance.
Upright Seated Posture on a Chair	Choose this basic stance if you have trouble sitting or kneeling on the floor.
Upright Seated Posture with Crossed Legs	This is a useful posture to start with because it allows you to adjust your pelvis and vertebrae.
Kneeling Postures	This posture and its variations are beneficial for some breathing techniques.
Standing Posture	While many yoga postures start from this standing basic stance, it can also be an asana (mountain posture).

Start to Gain Ground: Supine Postures

In this section, we show you the first set of modified postures and variations created to suit your needs after surgery. We have also included the reference postures so that you can see the differences and understand why and how the positions have been modified. Try different versions when your level of fitness is relatively good so that, during your rehabilitation or when you're less mobile, you'll know what works best for you. Be sure to choose the variation that best suits your current level of fitness, and don't hesitate to try out a prop if it helps you to enjoy the posture.

"Sometimes, when I was exhausted or absent minded, I was happy to just recline on the floor, feel my back on the floor, let my weight sink into the ground, relieve muscle tension, and become aware of my breath."

The supine postures presented here support stretching and muscle building and provide maximum safety and comfort when you are first starting your yoga practice. Activate your whole body while lying safely on the floor; as long as you feel the floor against the back of your body, you know you are well aligned.

Because our study was about women who had undergone breast surgery, we always started our yoga classes with supine postures. Due to the ongoing nature of the study, women whose surgeries had been performed just two or three days prior frequently joined the group—some even came in with drainage bottles still in their wounds! The supine postures offered a safe way for everyone in the group to start. Then, those who were comfortable and confident could slowly work up to more vigorous practice in the dynamic section of the class, where we moved in and out of a variety of standing and sitting postures. Finally, each class finished with relaxation, and everyone was able to compare how they felt mentally and physically after the class with how they had felt before.

Because of the number and variety of the postures, the contraindications and alignments are addressed in the detailed description of each asana.

SHANTI ASANA POSTURE

We recommend that you use a blanket or wear a jacket; it's much easier to relax when you feel warm.

Purposes

The first of our supine postures, shanti asana, familiarizes you with your own flexibility, makes you conscious of your breath, and relaxes you. The more you practice the posture, the better you will be at evaluating your body tone and the depth and rhythm of your breathing. Gradually, you will also become aware of your thoughts and feelings and begin to understand their influence on your temperament. Your general posture will also improve, your breathing will deepen, and you'll find it easier to become focused.

Contraindications

There are no contraindications for shanti asana. People with uncontrolled high blood pressure or ear and eye conditions should keep the head above heart level by resting it on a cushion or folded blanket while doing the postures. Jumping up suddenly out of the posture might lead to a decrease in blood pressure and make you feel dizzy. Slowly inhale while rolling upward into a standing posture or gently move into the next asana.

Alignments

In shanti asana, the spinal column between your tailbone and the crown of your head is stretched out. Consciously stretch your neck and lower your chin toward your chest. Relax your shoulder, face, and tongue muscles, and let your breath flow in and out through your nose.

In order to check for proper alignment and to become more conscious of your whole body, ask yourself the following questions: Is my neck stretched? Is my face relaxed? Are my tongue and larynx relaxed? Are both my shoulders and both my arms lying evenly on the ground? Which parts of my back are in contact with the floor? Which parts of my feet and legs touch the ground?

Lie on your back and stretch your entire spine.
Stretch your neck and lower your chin toward your sternum.
Close your eyes.
Relax your face and mouth muscles.
Relax your shoulders and make sure they lie flat on the floor.
Lay your arms beside your body, palms facing the ceiling.
Rotate your feet outward.
Breathe in and out deeply through your nose.

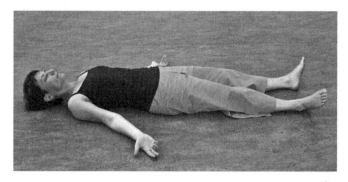

Variation with Cushion

If you have uncontrolled high blood pressure or ear and eye conditions, place your head on a folded blanket or cushion.

Variation with Bent Knees

If you suffer from acute pain in your lower back, bend your knees and place your feet on the floor. Keep them more than shoulder width apart, knees resting against each other. Relax fully.

DORSAL PALM TREE POSTURE

Although the dorsal palm tree posture is also a well-known standing posture that enhances your balance and flexibility, here we do the stretch lying on the back, as in shanti asana, but with arms out to each side.

Purposes

The modified dorsal palm tree posture done on the floor allows you to widen your chest and enlarge your breathing capacity. Your wrists and ankles gain flexibility through bending and stretching.

Contraindications

There are no contraindications for this modified version of the dorsal palm tree posture. If you suffer from uncontrolled high blood pressure or eye and ear conditions, keep your head above heart level by resting it on a cushion or folded blanket. Avoid suddenly exiting this posture, because the quick movement could lead to a decrease in blood pressure and make you feel dizzy. Slowly inhale while rolling upward or moving into the next asana.

Alignments

In the modified palm tree posture, stretch out your spine between your tailbone and the crown of your head. Don't forget to stretch your neck and lower your chin toward your sternum. Relax your shoulders, face, and tongue muscles, and let your breath flow in and out through your nose.

Part I

Get into the shanti asana, lying on your back with your body relaxed.

Consciously stretch your spine and flex your feet, with toes stretched toward your body.

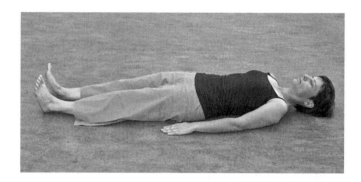

Place your hands on your belly with the tips of your middle fingers touching one another.

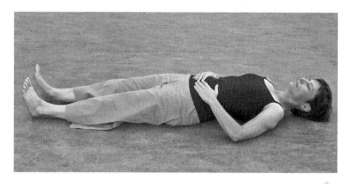

Inhale while opening your arms to the side, toward the floor. Touch the floor with the back of your hands if possible.

Exhale while moving your arms and hands back into the starting position.

Repeat the movement during at least six complete inhalations and exhalations.

Stop the movement and place your hands next to your body, palms facing down.

Feel the effects of the exercise.

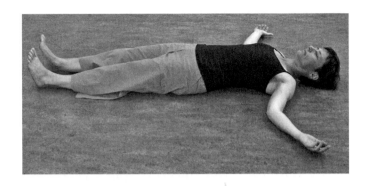

Part II

Inhale while pulling the balls of your feet closer to your body, without moving your legs. Make sure that your soles are stretched while your toes are bent back toward your body.

Exhale while stretching your feet toward the ground, toes out straight.

Repeat the movement during six complete inhalations and exhalations.

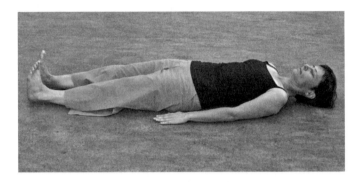

Part III

Continue the same movements, but now include your hands.

Inhale while flexing your feet toward your body and bending your hands up toward your arms.

Exhale while stretching your feet toward the ground and placing your hands on the ground.

Repeat the movement again during six complete inhalations and exhalations.

Feel the effects of the exercise.

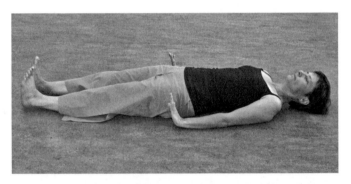

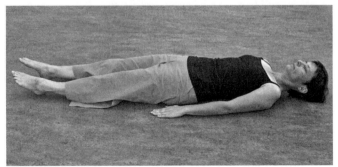

SUPINE TWIST POSTURE

The supine twist is a yoga posture well known to those who play sports. Used to strengthen the lower back and its connections to the pelvis, the supine twist can be done in a number of different ways.

Purposes

The modified version of the supine twist posture offers small and soothing movements, useful for those who suffer from lower back pain. The movements align the lower spine with the pelvis and, more importantly, keep the delicate sacroiliac joint flexible. The sacroiliac joint, which connects the sacrum, or lower end of the vertebrae, to the ilium or big pelvis bone, often blocks, becomes inflamed, and causes pain. The small movements of the modified supine twist posture can relieve this pain by increasing the joint's flexibility.

Contraindications

Women with breast cancer may encounter contraindications for this movement. In our study group, women suffering from metastasis in the sacrum either did not practice this posture or did so with great caution. If you're not sure whether you can do the posture, ask your therapist.

Alignments

Keep your spine stretched during the whole movement, and don't forget to stretch your neck and lower your chin toward your chest. If you suffer from uncontrolled high blood pressure or eye and ear conditions, rest your head on a cushion or folded blanket during the posture.

Proceed from the modified palm tree posture, or begin by lying on your back.

Stretch your spine and bend your knees.

Position the inner sides of your feet and knees close together.

Place your hands next to your body with your palms down on the floor.

Exhale while moving your closed knees and ankles gently to one side.

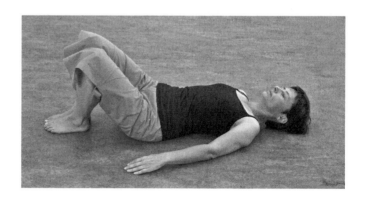

Inhale as you move your knees and ankles back to the center.

Exhale while moving your closed knees and ankles to the other side.

Inhale and move back to the middle.

Repeat the side-to-middle-to-side movement during at least six complete inhalations and exhalations.

Stop the movement, and place your hands next to your body, palms facing down.

Feel the effects of the exercise.

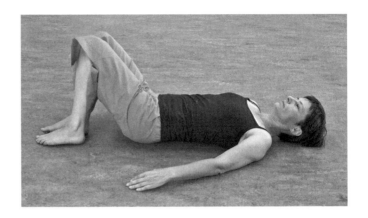

Reference Posture

In the full posture, lift your bent legs. Stretch both arms out at shoulder level. Keep your arms in this position throughout the exercise.

Lie on your back, bend both your knees, and place both your feet hip width apart on the floor.

Stretch out your arms at shoulder level, palms facing downward. Completely relax your shoulders and keep them on the floor. Slowly lift your knees toward your chest. Make sure that your neck is stretched and that both your lower legs and feet are relaxed.

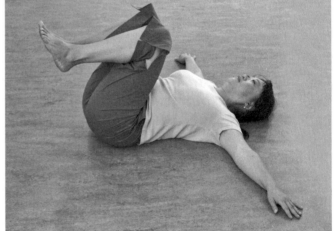

Exhale through your nose while moving your knees to the left and your head to the right. Start with small movements.

Inhale through your nose while moving your head and knees back into the middle.

Repeat the movement for six complete inhalations and exhalations. With each exhalation, make the movement bigger.

To continue the full asana from this position, place your feet back on the floor. Place your pelvis further to the right until your weight is on the left side of your bottom. Bend your knees again and lift them toward your chest.

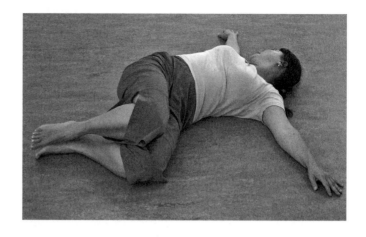

Exhale while moving the knees completely to the left side and your head to the right side. Make sure that both shoulders are still on the floor and that your neck is stretched. Rest your left hand on your right knee.

Maintain the posture for six complete inhalations and exhalations. You may close your eyes if you like. The more you relax, the easier it is to stay in this posture.

As you inhale turn back into the starting position and compare the feeling in both sides of your body: both legs, both sides of the pelvis, both sides of your shoulders, and your face.

Repeat the asana on the other side.

Finally, stretch out on your back and feel the effects of the complete asana.

HIP JOINT ROTATIONS

This is another gentle exercise that is very effective in preventing arthrosis. You can also do it easily in the morning while still lying in bed.

Purposes

Hip joint rotations enhance the mobility of your hip joints, open the pelvis, and improve your sitting postures. You will become aware of the differences in your legs and the mobility of your ankles, as well as of obstructions in your joints. If you hear popping and cracking noises, don't worry about it. Your body is simply telling you that you're not used to the movement. The noise may be caused by roughness on the surface of the cartilage or gas formation in the fluid between joints.

Contraindications

People who have just undergone hip replacement surgery should not do this posture. If you have had breast cancer surgery, be careful to choose the correct radius of movement. For best results, start with small movements and gradually expand them over the course of the exercise.

Alignments

Once again, keep your spine stretched, lower your chin toward your chest, and rest your head on a cushion or folded blanket if you suffer from uncontrolled high blood pressure or eye and ear conditions.

Proceed from the modified supine twist posture, or begin by lying on your back.

Stretch your spine and bend your knees.

Place both of your feet hip width apart on the floor. Stretch your arms out to the side, palms facing up. Stretch your neck, lower your chin toward your chest, and relax your face and mouth muscles.

Inhale while stretching out your left leg.

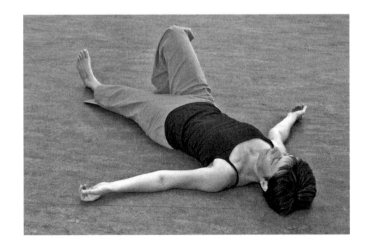

Lift your leg and, in a continuous leg movement, circle to the left, parallel to the floor. Start with small movements and widen the angle only when you feel comfortable doing so.

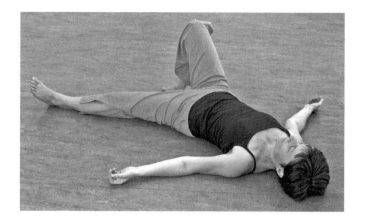

Exhale while bending your left knee and move back into the starting position.

Repeat the movement for six complete inhalations and exhalations.

Then, still with your left leg, change the direction of the circular movement.

Inhale while rotating your left knee to the left and stretching your left leg, making a circular movement.

Exhale while bending your left leg and moving it back into the starting position.

Repeat the movement during six complete inhalations and exhalations.

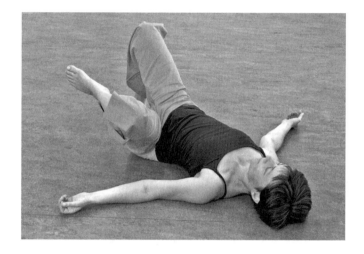

Place both feet on the ground and compare the feeling in each leg, both sides of your pelvis, and both sides of your face. Feel the polarity of your body, in this case, how the left side feels compared to the right.

Continue to the other side and repeat the exercise with your right leg.

Finally, lie on your back and feel the effects of the complete exercise.

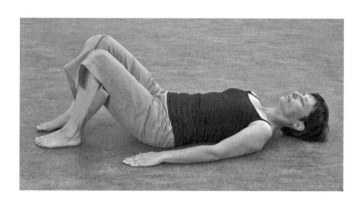

DORSAL TREE POSTURE

This yoga posture improves your balance. In the full posture you must be able to rotate your bent knee to the side; in this modified version, you move safely while lying on your back.

Purposes

Designed to enhance the mobility of the hip joints, this exercise also opens the pelvis and improves your positioning in all sitting postures. After exercising on one side, you might feel a difference in your legs regarding shape and height—the trained leg and hip feel bigger and seem to be resting on a higher level than the untrained leg.

Contraindications

To safely complete this exercise, relax your legs without hurting your hip joints or lifting your lower back. You might find that placing your bent knee on a cushion or folded blanket is helpful.

Alignments

As in all of the previously mentioned supine postures, stretch your spine and lower your chin toward your chest. If you suffer from uncontrolled high blood pressure or eye and ear conditions, rest your head on a cushion.

Proceed from the hip joint rotation exercise, or begin by lying on your back.

Consciously stretch your spine. Stretch your neck, lower your chin toward your chest, and relax your face and mouth muscles.

Bend your knees and place both your feet hip width apart on the floor. Lay your arms close to the sides of your body, palms facing downward.

Exhale as you lower your left knee to the side. If it helps you to completely relax your whole leg, place a cushion under your knee.

With the next exhalation, stretch your right leg. Flex your right foot with your toes stretched back toward your body. Touch the inner side of your right knee with the sole of your left foot.

Hold the posture during six complete inhalations and exhalations.

Inhale while bending your right knee and placing your right foot back on the floor.

With another inhalation, lift your left knee and return to the starting position, feet hip width apart.

Compare the feeling in each of your legs, hip joints, shoulders, and sides of your face.

Continue to the other side, holding the posture for six complete inhalations and exhalations.

Finally, lie on your back and feel the effects of the completed exercise.

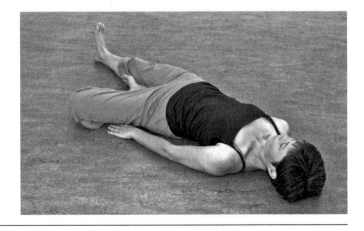

DORSAL KNEE ROTATIONS

Most people only notice their knee joints when they hurt. Knee rotations help you properly align your knee joints and prevent knee problems.

Purposes

The easy-to-do dorsal knee rotations align the delicate knee joints while you are in a safe posture, which is very helpful for people with knee problems. During the exercise, you will feel gentle movements in your knees and become aware of obstructions and noises.

Contraindications

If you have knee replacements, consult with your therapist. Perform this exercise with care, controlling the movement and being careful not to swing your lower legs around. Gradually, the strength of your leg muscles will increase. Start with small movements and expand them over the course of the exercise.

Alignments

Stretch your spine and lower your chin toward your chest. As always, if you suffer from uncontrolled high blood pressure or eye and ear conditions rest your head on a cushion or folded blanket. Exercise with slow movements.

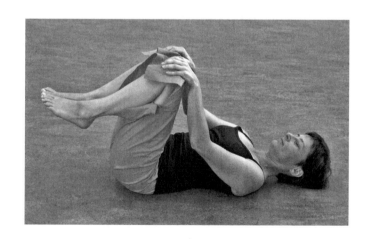

Proceed from the tree posture or begin by lying on your back.

Consciously stretch your spine. Stretch your neck, lower your chin toward your chest, and relax your face and mouth muscles.

Bend your knees and pull them close to your chest.

Place your right hand on your right knee and your left hand on your left knee.

Slowly start moving your lower legs in small circles. As you proceed, listen to the noises made by your joins (ankles, knees, and hips). Feel the obstructions.

Repeat the movement during six complete inhalations and exhalations.

Continue the exercise rotating in the opposite direction. Compare the noises you hear and the obstructions you feel during the movements to those from the first side.

Finally, lie on your back and feel the effects of the exercise.

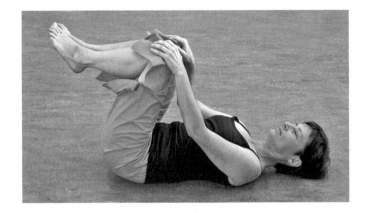

KNEES TO CHEST

Knees to chest is another posture that can also easily be done while lying in bed—in the morning to gently stretch your back, in the evening to prepare for a relaxing sleep.

Purposes

The knees to chest posture deepens your breath. At the same time, it stretches your lower back and bends it toward the belly, widening the spaces between the vertebrae of the lower back.

Contraindications

Knees to chest is a very gentle posture and is only harmful to someone who suffers from abdominal pain.

Alignments

It is vital to synchronize your breathing with your movement. Think of inhaling as raising your abdominal wall and extending the space and movement, and moving your knees makes space for the belly. Think of exhaling as lowering your abdominal wall and reducing the space of your belly, allowing your knees to come closer to your chest.

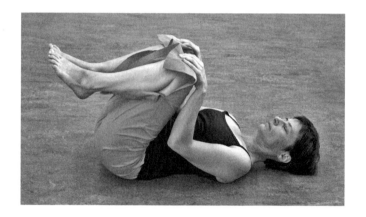

Proceed from the knee rotating posture or begin by lying on your back.

Consciously stretch your spine. Stretch your neck, lower your chin toward your chest, and relax your face and mouth muscles.

Bend your knees and pull them to your chest.

Place your right hand on your right knee and your left hand on your left knee. Make sure that both your lower legs and feet are relaxed and that your neck is stretched.

Exhale through your nose, bend your arms, and pull your knees closer to your chest.

Inhale through your nose, stretch your arms, and move your knees away from your chest.

Repeat the movement through at least six complete inhalations and exhalations.

Place your feet back on the floor and feel the effects of the movement. Close your eyes if you like.

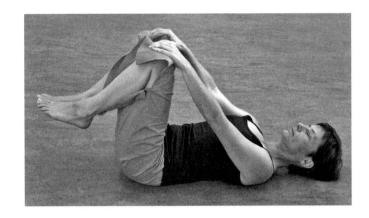

Variation

Perform the knee to the chest posture with one knee at a time. Place both feet on the floor, and then bring one knee close to your chest.

Inhale while you extend the space between belly and knee; exhale while you reduce the space. After you have practiced with one knee, place both feet on the floor and compare the feeling in both legs, both sides of your pelvis, and both sides of your face. Feel the polarity of your body. Now repeat the exercise with your other knee.

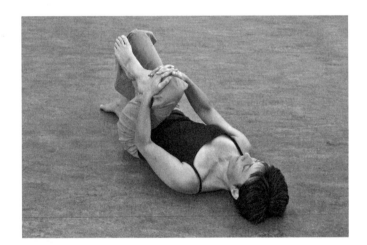

LEGS AND ARMS STRETCH

Though this posture may seem easy, it actually takes a lot of strength in your belly and leg muscles. After a period of exercising, you will tell the difference.

Purposes

By performing the leg stretch, you will get a good sense of the flexibility and strength of your leg and abdominal muscles. You will also feel how the muscles of your legs, back, and belly coordinate. Become aware of the mobility of your shoulder joints, and learn to tighten and relax the muscles of your neck, shoulders, and arms.

Remember

After breast surgery, it is vital to exercise hands, arms, and shoulders. If your lymph nodes have been removed, it becomes especially important because nerve injury to the shoulder and back muscles can lead to lymphedema or fluid retention that causes swelling of the tissue. Exercising the hands, arms, and shoulders supports the transport of tissue fluid back into the circulatory system. Do the arm and shoulder postures regularly during the day and in your yoga class. (See chapters 6 and 7 and part III for more postures.)

Contraindications

If you suffer from abdominal pain, exercise with caution and consult your therapist.

Alignments

In this exercise, your breathing supports the movement. Gently stretch your arms and legs, being careful not to fully stretch your arms and knees in the beginning. You may also choose to practice with one arm or one leg at a time when you first start. Your arms and legs will stretch after exercising regularly for a while.

Proceed from the knee to chest posture, or begin by lying on your back.

Consciously stretch your spine. Stretch your neck, lower your chin toward your chest, and relax your face and mouth muscles.

Bend your knees and pull them to your chest.

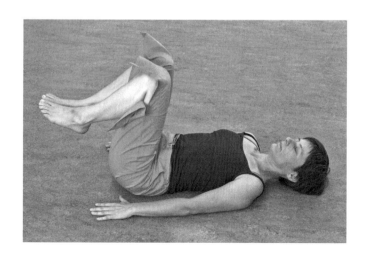

Part I

Place your arms and hands beside your body, palms facing down.

Inhale through your nose while stretching your legs upward. The soles of your feet should be parallel to the ceiling.

Exhale while bending your legs back into the starting position.

Repeat the stretching and bending of your legs during six complete inhalations and exhalations.

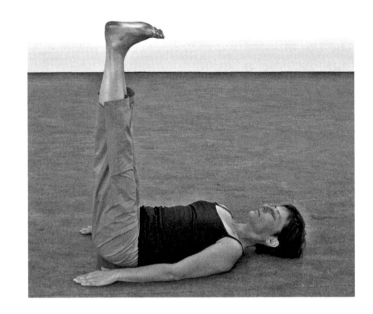

Part II

Keep your legs stretched and the soles of your feet parallel to the ceiling.

Inhale through your nose while lifting your arms upward.

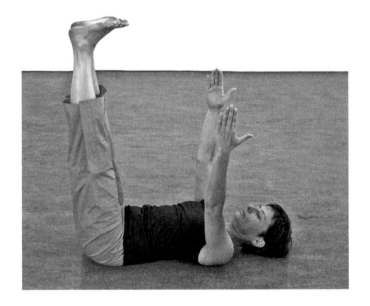

With your arms still up, alternate between lifting your right shoulder and your left shoulder up from the floor and lowering it back down.

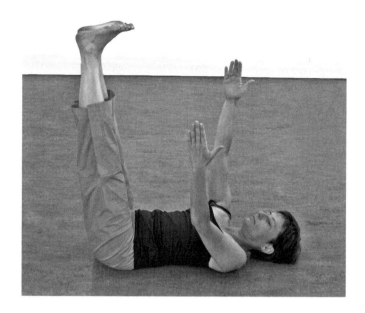

Keep to a steady breathing rhythm that matches the pace of your movements.

Repeat the movement of your right and left shoulder six times on each side.

As you exhale, lower your arms to the floor.

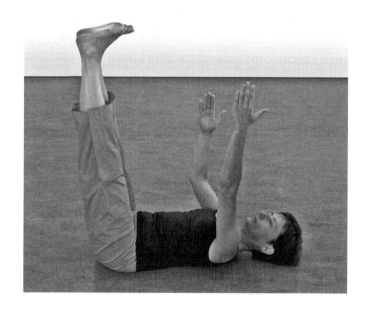

Variation

While arms are up, open and close your hands (pumping).
Repeat the movement during six inhalations and exhalations.
As you exhale, lower your arms.
Feel the effect of the exercise. Close your eyes if it feels good to do so.

Reference Posture

During this exercise, fully stretch your arms and legs.

Inhale through your nose while stretching your legs upward and bringing your arms down straight on the floor above your head.

Exhale while getting back into the starting position.

Repeat the movement during six complete inhalations and exhalations.

Finally, lie on your back and feel the effects of the exercise. You may close your eyes if you like.

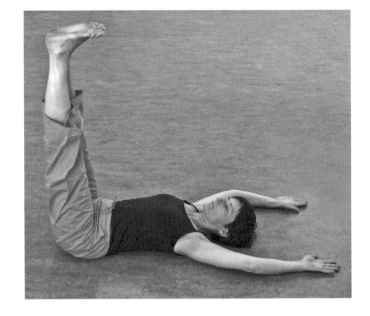

DORSAL LION POSTURE

Often used as a mood booster, we use the lion posture for stretching and strengthening.

Purposes

Lion posture, the last of the supine postures in this chapter, is a modified version of a classic yoga posture. When done in a supine position, it strengthens your neck and shoulder muscles. It works well against a double chin. Additionally, this yoga posture is known to help lift your mood.

Contraindications

If you have pain in your neck and shoulders, perform this exercise with great caution and consult with your therapist.

Alignments

During all the previous postures, you inhale and exhale through your nose. This is the first exception. You exhale vigorously through your mouth and put out your tongue.

Proceed from the modified dorsal leg and arm stretch, or begin by lying on your back.

Consciously stretch your spine. Stretch your neck, lower your chin toward your chest, and relax your face and mouth muscles.

Bend your knees and place your feet hip width apart from each other.

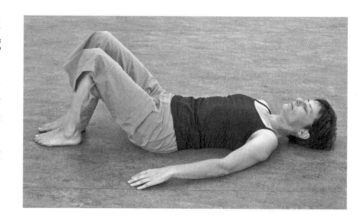

Inhale while lifting your shoulders off the ground.

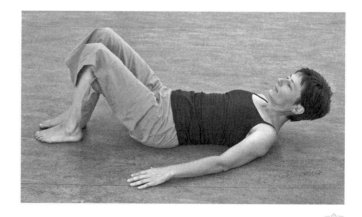

Exhale and put out your tongue making a loud "haaa" sound.

Bring your tongue back in and lower your torso.

Repeat the exercise three times.

After the third time, maintain the position with your torso lifted for another three complete inhalations and exhalations.

As you exhale, lower your torso.

Rub your hands forcefully together until you feel their warmth.

Stretch your neck muscles with your hands by gently moving your hands from the shoulders upward to your head on both sides of your spine.

Finally, stop the action, stretch your legs, lie on your back, and feel the effects of the exercise. You may close your eyes if you like.

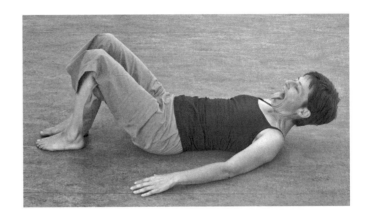

Reference Posture

Sit on the floor with your sit bones resting on your heels. Stretch your feet, tops flat on the floor and toes pointed inward.

Pull your pelvis into an upright position, tighten your pelvic muscles, and relax your belly.

Straighten your spinal column, and raise your sternum.

Relax your shoulders and arms, and rest your hands on your thighs.

Align your chin parallel to the ground, and relax your face, lips, and tongue.

Breathe in and out deeply through your nose.

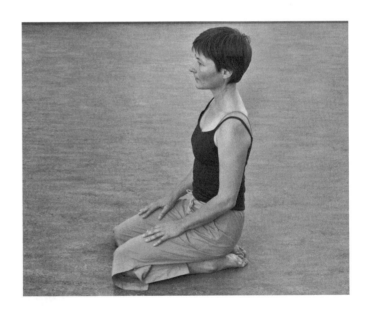

As you exhale, move your torso and arms forward until your hands rest like claws on your knees. Exhale through your mouth, extending your tongue out as far as you can and opening your eyes wide, roaring "aaaah."

Return to the starting position with an inhalation.

Take a rest for two complete breaths.

Repeat the exercise three times.

Rest on your heels, close your eyes, and feel the effects.

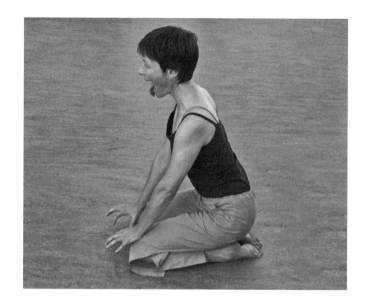

QUICK LOOK

Chapter 7 START TO GAIN GROUND: SUPINE POSTURES	
Shanti Asana Posture	Helps you become familiar with your flexibility.
Dorsal Palm Tree Posture	Allows you to widen your chest and enlarge your breathing capacity.
Supine Twist Posture	A very effective exercise for all who suffer from pain in the lower spine.
Hip Joint Rotations	Enhances the mobility of your hip joints.
Dorsal Tree Posture	Opens the pelvis and improves all sitting postures.
Dorsal Knee Rotations	Easy to do and aligns bones and ligaments of the knee joints.
Knees to Chest	Deepens the breath and widens the spaces between the vertebrae of the lower back.
Legs and Arms Stretch	Vital after the removal of lymph nodes as it supports the transport of tissue fluid back into the circulation, and increases flexibility and strength of leg and abdominal muscles.
Dorsal Lion Posture	Strengthens neck and shoulder muscles, fights a double chin, and is known to improve mood

8

Stretch and Breathe: Pranayama Postures

One of the main goals of yoga is to influence physical and mental well-being via breathing. Synchronizing breathing and movement is paramount, and every asana is accompanied by breathing techniques. Because the techniques help you to get into and maintain each yoga posture, we have provided detailed instructions on breathing during each movement and stance. When you are able to concentrate on your breathing and movement and realize how it affects you, you gain strength and self-awareness.

Conscious breathing that is not only an important part of an asana but an exercise in itself is called pranayama. These exercises are done in still postures, either lying or sitting on the floor, or with the aid of a simple movement. For women who have just had breast cancer surgery, breathing techniques are particularly vital because they deepen the breath and stretch the group of muscles responsible for widening and narrowing the chest. Pranayama postures can also stimulate circulation or digestion, can tell you about the actual condition of your body, and, depending on which pranayama exercises you are doing, can influence diverse sections of the breathing apparatus, such as the diaphragm, rib cage, or bronchi. In addition, breathing techniques also increase the oxygen level in the blood, and the circulation of oxygen-rich blood increases your muscle power as well as your mental power.

Finally, pranayama helps to relieve inner tensions and enables you to mentally relax.

> *"I practice some of the postures we did during the yoga class at home by myself, especially those from the pranayama section."*

Breathing techniques play a key role in helping you get focused, concentrate, and meditate. At the end of every exercise in this book you will find instructions to "feel the effect." While it may not seem like it, this is an essential part of each exercise because if you cannot feel the effects, you cannot learn to actively achieve balance and stability. Being aware of progress and regress is essential to learning and developing.

> *"Yoga also improved my singing. I am a singer in a choir, and we do breathing exercises before we sing. Yoga breathing exercises are especially good for singers."*

A good way to improve focus and concentratation is to consciously breathe while moving. If you can influence your posture as well as your mind via breathing, you will not only perform better at yoga but will also better manage your illness, therapy, and rehabilitation—both physically and mentally.

> *"Well, breathing and making noises was difficult for me at the beginning. I had trouble doing it. But I tried it out and noticed the effect on my ability to concentrate and relax. Conscious breathing enhanced my posture while standing."*

Contraindications

Don't underestimate the effects of yoga breathing techniques. Though there are only a few contraindications, you should immediately stop a yoga breathing exercise if it doesn't feel right and return to your normal inhalation and exhalation.

Alignments

The regular breath in yoga is a nostril breath, but in rare cases other methods, such as exhaling through the mouth, will be indicated. The breath initiates and leads the movement, so if you feel short of breath, slow down the pace of the movement. More information is given with each posture.

Note:

The exercises in this and the following section can also be done sitting on a chair, stool, or cushion (see chapter 1 "Upright Seated Postures" for more information).

DETOX BREATHING

What is "detox" breathing? Through vigorous exhalation, you let off steam. Breath you might have held onto is released as tensions you might unconsciously suffer from are relieved.

If you continue from lion posture, roll your body over to one side to get up, and move into the kneeling posture. Otherwise, sit with your sit bones on your heels. Pull your pelvis into an upright position, stretch your spine, and lower your chin toward your sternum.

Relax your shoulders, arms, face, and tongue muscles.

Place your hands on top of your thighs.

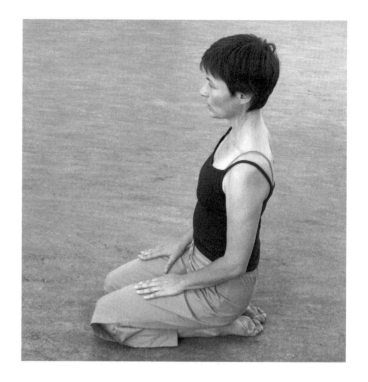

Inhale through your nose.

Purse your lips and clench your teeth, drawing in your belly as you lean forward, and exhale three times making the sound "shh." (Do not inhale or let any air flow in between exhalations.)

Inhale, stretch out your neck and raise your stretched out torso until you are back in the starting position.

Repeat the exercise three times.

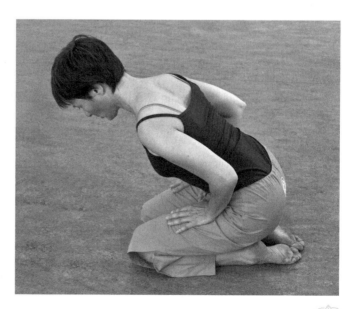

After the third time, remain leaning forward, and place your forearms on the floor.

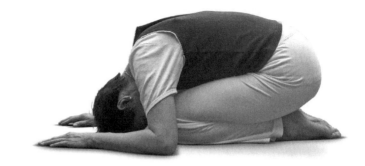

You can also place your forearms on your knees.

Bow your head.

Maintain the position for three complete inhalations. With each exhalation, relax your shoulders toward the floor. With each inhalation, feel the stretch of your spine.

With a final inhalation, stretch your spine and raise your stretched torso back into the starting position.

Keep your eyes closed and feel the effect of the pranayama exercise.

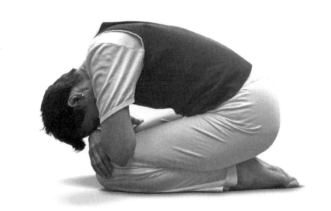

Variation on a Chair

You can do this pranayama exercise sitting on a chair.

Sit down on a chair. Place your feet hip width apart. Align your knee joints above your ankles, pull your pelvis upright, stretch your spine, extend the crown of your head upward, and lower your chin toward your sternum. Place your hands on top of your thighs and start the movement. Purse your lips and clench your teeth, drawing in your belly as you lean forward, and exhale three times making the sound "shh." After the third time rest your forearms on your knees.

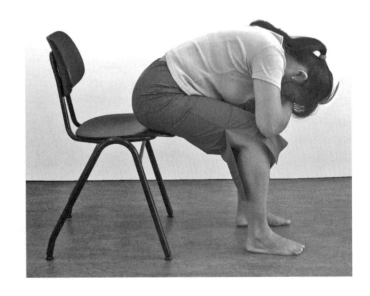

In the full detox breathing posture, you rest by placing your head on the floor in front of your knees. Lay your arms beside your body, palms facing upward.

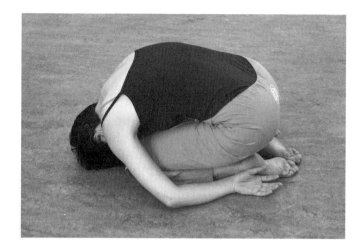

Note:

The forward bend with your arms or hands resting on the floor or on your thighs is a posture in itself, called the "folded leaf posture." If you ever need a break, or just want to stretch your back or relax your shoulders, get into this posture.

Reference Posture

As you inhale, come back into the starting posture. As you exhale, bend backward. Place your hands behind your back with the fingertips pointing to your feet.

Make sure that your knees are close together and still resting on the floor.

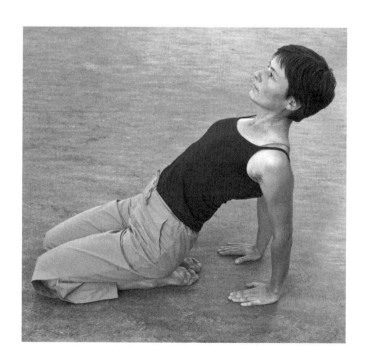

CAMEL POSTURE

The camel posture widens your chest, strengthens your shoulder and arm muscles, flexes the back, and expands your breathing space. If you exercise in the kneeling posture, you also strengthen your thigh and belly muscles. During our study, this was one of the most loved exercises.

Continue from the detox breathing posture or move into the kneeling posture.

Inhale while rising up on your knees, pointing your toes, and opening your arms to the side. Make sure your thighs are in an upright position and push your pubic bone forward.

Exhale and return to the starting position.

Repeat the movement for six complete inhalations and exhalations.

To do the whole asana, maintain the posture with opened arms for three complete inhalations and exhalations.

As you exhale, return to the kneeling posture and feel the effects of the exercise.

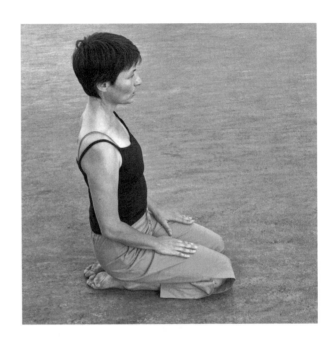

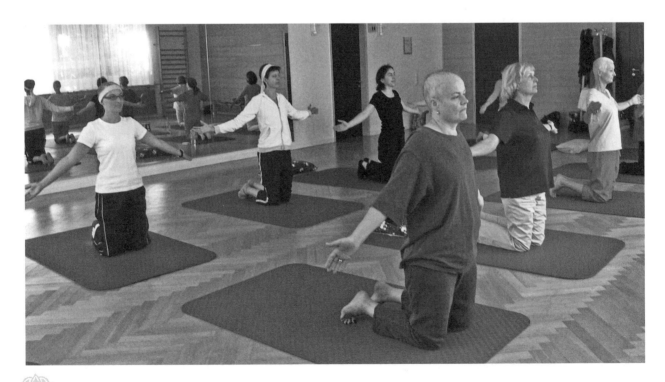

Variation on a Chair

You can also perform this pranayama exercise sitting on a chair, which lets you rest your legs and work with your torso and arms.

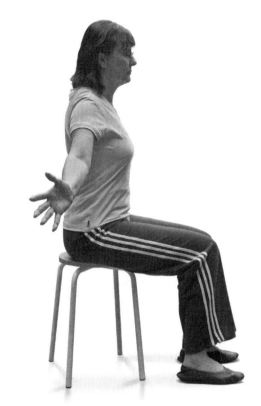

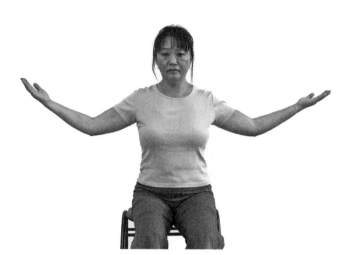

Reference Posture

If you have enough flexibility to bend backward, you can place your hands on your heels. As you inhale, rise to your knees while simultaneously doing a backward circle with each arm, one after the other, and grasp your heels. Maintain the position for six complete inhalations and exhalations.

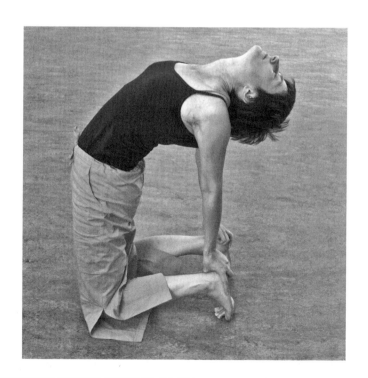

TIGER BREATHING

The tiger breathing exercise enhances your awareness of your spine. If you are able to bend and stretch your spine consciously, you can check your posture during the day. The exercise also synchronizes breathing and movement.

Note:

After surgery it is important that you exercise gently. Make sure your arms can hold the weight of your torso.

Continue from the camel posture or move into the kneeling posture.

As you inhale, bend forward, keeping your arms straight, until your hands touch the floor.

Make sure that your wrists are under your shoulders and that your knees are under your hip joints. These alignments help you to exercise without hurting your joints.

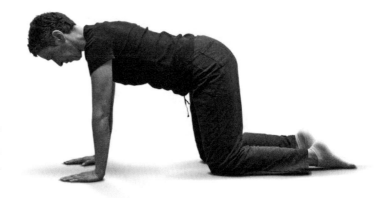

Exhale as you bend or curl your spine upward, vertebra by vertebra, starting at your tailbone and moving all the way up through the lumbar, thoracic, and cervical spine. Bow your head at the end.

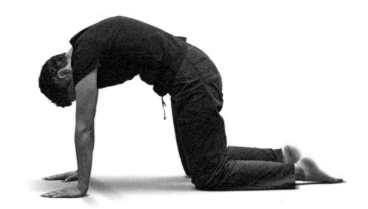

Inhale and stretch your spine downward, vertebra by vertebra, starting at your tailbone and moving all the way up through the lumbar, thoracic, and cervical spine. Lift your head at the end.

Repeat the bend and stretch exercise for six complete inhalations and exhalations.

Inhale and get back into the kneeling posture. Place your fingers on top of your thighs and relax. Feel the effects. Close your eyes if you like.

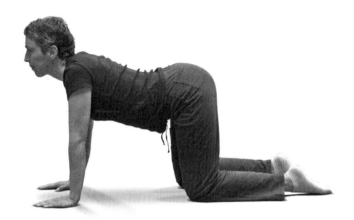

Variation on a Chair

You can do the tiger breathing exercise sitting on a chair. Start the exercise with your hands placed on top of your knees.

Exhale, round your back, and bow your head.

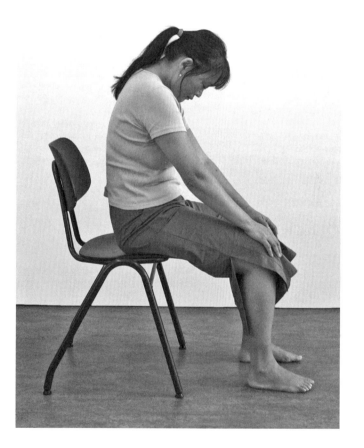

Inhale, stretch your back, and raise your head.

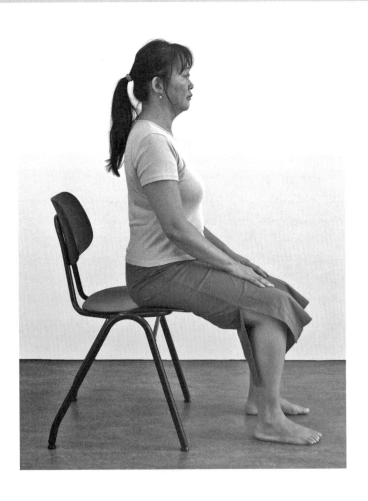

QUICK LOOK

Chapter 8 STRETCH AND BREATHE: PRANAYAMA POSTURES	
Detox Breathing	Vigorous exhalation allows you to let off steam; it releases the breath and relieves tensions.
Camel Posture	Widens the chest and expands the breathing space, strengthens shoulder and arm muscles, flexes the back.
Tiger Breathing	Enhances the awareness of the spine and synchronizes breathing and movement.

9

Relieve Tensions: Postures for Neck, Shoulders, and Arms

After surgery, your instinct is to re-duce the movement of your arms in order to protect the wound, and you might tend to hold one or both arms closer to your torso. After a short time this caution is un-necessary, but, forgetting that your shoulders are tight and pulled up, you might continue carrying yourself that way. As a result, your shoulders will hurt because of this increased tension and you might even develop a headache. Thinking that the pain is from the wound, you continue to hold yourself in the posture.

To break this vicious cycle, exercise your neck, shoulder, and arm muscles regularly. Pay close attention to this important section.

Contraindications and alignments are described for each posture.

ARM AND HEAD COORDINATION

This exercise develops your ability to coordinate head and arm movements. At the same time, you learn to synchronize movement and breathing and increase your ability to focus.

Continue from the tiger breathing posture or move into the kneeling posture. You can also perform this exercise sitting on a chair, as shown.

Sit with your sit bones on your heels. Pull your pelvis upright, stretch your spine, and lower your chin toward your sternum. Relax your shoulders and arms, along with your face and tongue muscles.

Place your hands on top of your thighs.

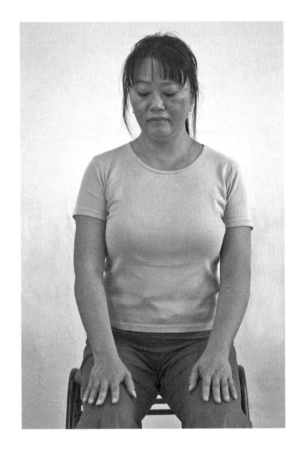

As you inhale, move your right hand to the right side at shoulder height and follow the movement with your eyes.

Look into your right palm as you would look into a mirror.

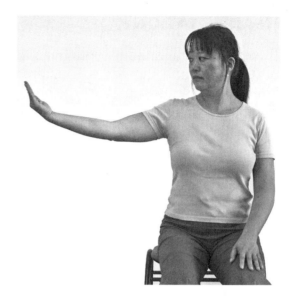

Exhale while moving your right hand to your left shoulder and follow the movement with your eyes.

Inhale and again move your right arm to the side and follow the movement with your eyes, again looking into your palm as you would a mirror.

Exhale and move your right arm back to your right thigh.

Continue the exercise, moving your left hand to the left side.

Repeat the exercise six times.

Finally, return to the starting posture and feel the effects in your arms and shoulders. Keep your eyes closed if you like.

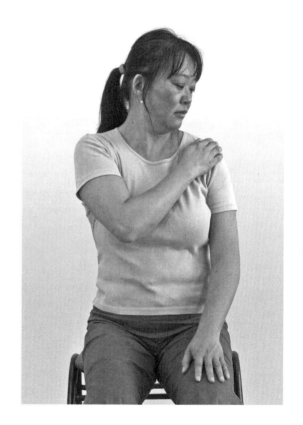

HEAD ROTATIONS

If you sit in a car and turn your head to see behind you, you can immediately tell the fitness of your neck and shoulders. To maintain or regain the mobility of your joints and the flexibility of your muscles, practice these neck, shoulder, and arm postures. They are regular exercises in a yoga class and can be done easily, so you should practice them occasionally during the day.

Note:

You can turn your head, rotate it, bow it, and shake it. Do each possible joint movement separately so that you are gentle with your joints, exercise safely, and train your awareness for all head movements.

Continue from the arms and head movement, or move into a kneeling or a seated posture.

As you inhale, stretch your spinal column and neck.

Exhale and relax your shoulders.

Keep your chin parallel to the floor, and make sure that your head does not bow and your shoulders stay relaxed.

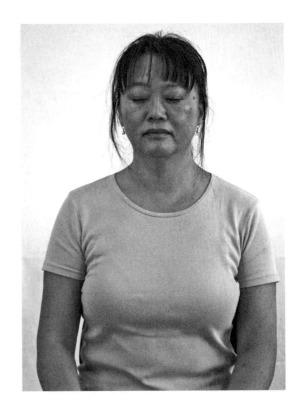

Inhale while turning your head to the right.

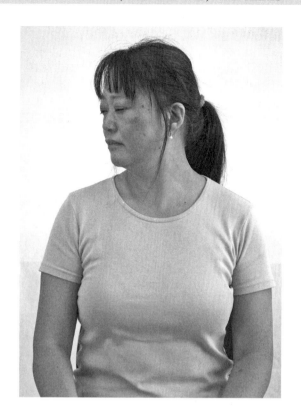

Exhale while turning your head to the left without bowing.

Repeat the rotation for six complete inhalations and exhalations.

Get back into your initial posture. Feel the effect of the rotations. You may close your eyes if you like.

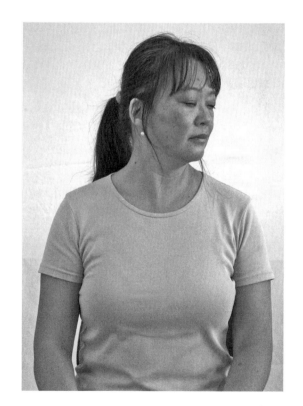

HEAD BOW SIDEWAYS

The head bow sideways is important because it exercises the muscles of your neck and shoulders. While performing this posture, make sure that you keep both shoulders in a relaxed position.

Note:

Make sure that your shoulders are relaxed and that your head does not turn and bow at the same time.

Continue from the head rotation movement, or move into a kneeling or seated position.

As you inhale, stretch your spinal column and neck, and relax your shoulders.

While exhaling, gently bow your head to the right side, moving your right ear closer to your shoulder. Make sure that both your shoulders stay relaxed.

As you inhale, slowly raise your head into the starting position.

Exhale and gently bow your head to the left side.

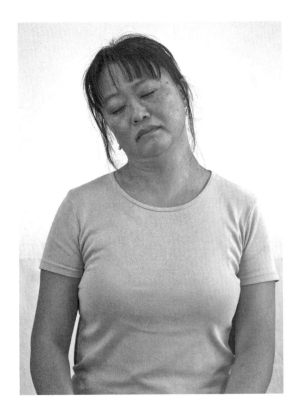

As you inhale, slowly raise your head into the starting position.

Repeat the movements for six complete inhalations and exhalations, three movements per side.

Finally, get back into the initial posture and feel the effect of the stretches. You may close your eyes if you like.

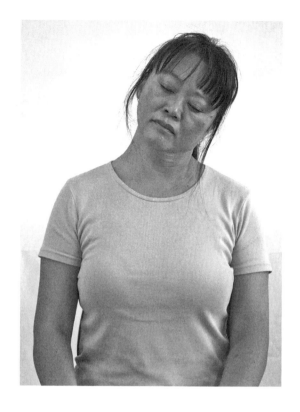

HEAD BOW FORWARD

In the next step, you lower your head forward and stretch your shoulder and neck muscles.

Continue from the head bow sideways movement, or move into a kneeling or seated posture.

As you inhale, stretch your spinal column and neck and relax your shoulders.

While exhaling, gently bow your head forward to the right until your chin gets close to your chest. Make sure that both your shoulders stay relaxed.

As you inhale, slowly raise your head into the starting position.

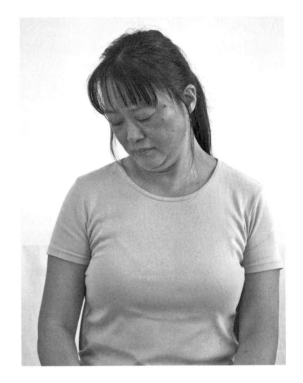

Exhale and gently bow your head forward and to the left.

As you inhale, slowly raise your head into the starting position.

Repeat the movements for six complete inhalations and exhalations, three movements on each side.

Finally, return to your initial posture and feel the effect of the stretches. You may close your eyes if you like.

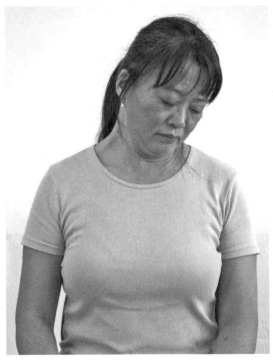

QUICK LOOK

Chapter 9 RELIEVE TENSIONS: POSTURES FOR NECK, SHOULDERS, AND ARMS	
Arm and Head Coordination	Develops the ability to coordinate head and arm movement, to synchronize movement and breathing, and to focus.
Head Rotations	Done one direction at a time, and help in maintaining or re-gaining the mobility of joints and the flexibility of neck and shoulder muscles.
Head Bow Sideways	
Head Bow Forward	

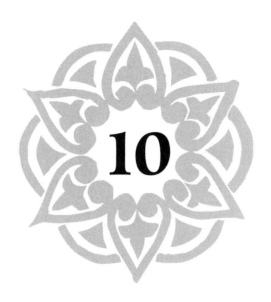

10

Pay Attention: Eye Exercises

With a stretched spine and relaxed neck and shoulder muscles, you are primed for the next set of yoga postures: eye exercises. Though you may not realize it, you can train your eye muscles in the same way that you can train other muscle groups. Yoga exercises for the eyes help you maintain good eye sight and can also provide relief for burning and itching eyes. For cancer patients, these exercises are important in alleviating the vision problems that chemotherapy can cause.

Exercising your eyes for just a couple of minutes each day enables your ocular muscles to better adapt to the loss of flexibility that happens as we age, helps your eyes remain moist, increases blood circulation, and relaxes the eye. You will find that the relaxation gained through this exercise will improve your vision.

Contraindications

If you normally wear glasses, take them off during these exercises. If you have serious eye problems, such as glaucoma or macular degeneration, you should talk to your doctor first.

FOCUS NEAR AND FAR

If your eyes are constantly focusing at the same distance (reading, watching TV, working at the computer), your eye muscles weaken in the same way that a constant seated position weakens your leg and belly muscles. Most people fail to realize that eye muscles, like any other muscle, need a workout to stay flexible and maintain strength.

The next exercises actively alternate your focus on close and distant objects. By moving your arms at the same time, you also increase muscle strength.

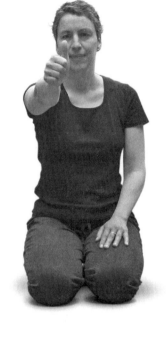

Continue from the head bow forward exercise, or move into the kneeling or seated posture.

Extend one arm to eye level, make a fist, and put up your thumb.

Look at the tip of your nose and take a breath in and out.

Look at your thumbnail and breathe in and out.

Look at an object that is close by, and breathe in and out.

Look at an object in the distance, and breathe in and out.

With the next inhalation, you no longer lock your eyes onto an object. Instead, just look into the sky or ahead of you and breathe out again.

Repeat each step in reverse order until you are looking at your nose again.

Do the exercise six times. Change to the other arm if you like.

At the end, put your arms on top of your thighs.

Close your eyes before you continue with the next exercise.

Note:

This exercise can be done discretely during the day. Instead of looking at your thumbnail, choose an object near you to look at.

"I was impressed that a yoga class also encompassed a set of eye exercises. Since we had wonderful trees in front of our windows, it was a treat to do the near and distant focus exercise during class."

"The exercises helped me overcome my blurred vision, but it was exhausting for my arms."

THE LYING EIGHT

During the first eye exercise, you switched back and forth between focusing on something close and focusing on something far. With the next exercise, you train your peripheral vision. Done together with arm movement and proper breathing, eye exercises can also help you to strengthen your arm muscles and help you better concentrate.

Continue from the focus near and far exercise, or move into the kneeling or seated posture.

Extend your right arm to eye level, make a fist, and put up your thumb.

Focus on your thumbnail with both eyes. As you do this exercise, hold your head in a fixed position, and move only your eyes as you focus on and follow the movements of your thumb.

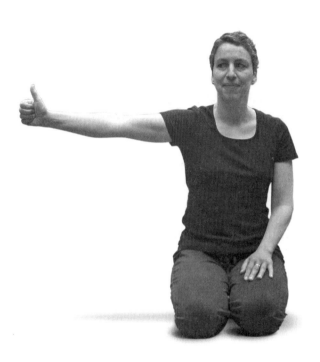

Start moving your right hand and thumb upward as far as possible, making sure that you can still see your thumbnail. Continue moving your hand completely to the right, staying focused on the thumbnail at all times. Follow your thumb as your stretched right arm moves downward along the lower right half of your peripheral vision, and then proceed back to the starting position.

Lower your right arm, and bring your left arm up. Do the same exercise to the left side.

Repeat the exercise twice to each side.

Close your eyes, and continue on to the following exercise.

CUPPING AND BLINKING

During the two preceding eye exercises, your eyes were wide open and the muscles active. The next exercise supports the relaxation of your eyes and facial muscles, and the blinking helps moisten your eyes.

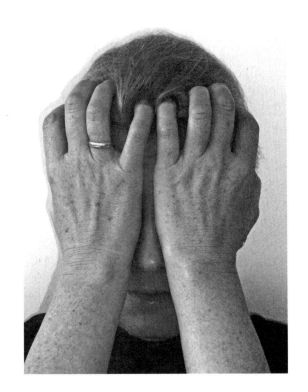

While your eyes are closed, rub your hands forcefully together until you feel their warmth.

Completely cover your closed eyes with your palms, and let your fingertips rest on your hair line. Feel the warmth of your palms being transferred, and completely relax your eyes.

Hold the posture for as long as you can feel the warmth of your palms.

While keeping your eyes closed, remove your hands, and relax your arms in your lap.

Start blinking your eyes, quickly at first and then slowly.

Finally, open your eyes and keep them open. Relax your whole body and feel the effects.

QUICK LOOK

Chapter 10 PAY ATTENTION: EYE EXERCISES	
Focus Near and Far	Trains eye muscles by alternating tightening and relaxing.
The Lying Eight	Increases peripheral vision.
Cupping and Blinking	Relaxes eye and facial muscles and moistens the eyes.

Back to Old Heights: Standing Postures

With the next set of yoga asanas, practiced during the dynamic portion of the class, you build muscles from your feet to your arms. Breathing and moving correctly are essential to getting into the postures and holding them. The exercises shown here are demanding but also very energizing, relieving energy loss as they boost your circulation and strengthen the muscles that help you stay balanced. The changes between forward and backward bends and among side bends, rotations, and balancing postures are not only good variations, but will make you aware of all the different movements and capabilities of your body.

Along with these physical benefits, the energy of the asanas promotes your mental well-being, and yoga asanas such as the hero postures make you feel your strength, get focused, and gain courage.

"Depending on my mood and well-being, I prefer different postures. When I feel very energetic I love to do the hero postures. I feel my muscle strength and bring my energy to the posture."

After surgery, many women tend to hunch their shoulders, tightening the chest, rounding the upper back, and moving the head and chin forward. Such poor posture hurts the upper spine in many ways and causes shallow breathing. In order to counter this, you must regularly practice stretching and pulling the shoulders backward and sitting upright. We helped women do this during our yoga classes by exercising the neck, shoulder, and arm muscles in all postures: lying, sitting, and standing.

For example, the head and eye exercises were done sitting upright. Here, we focus on the standing versions.

Contraindications and Alignments

Because of the high number and great variety of the postures, we address the contraindications and alignments in the detailed description of each asana.

HERO I

This modified posture, in which you open your arms to the side, is a good start after surgery. Like the reference posture in which you stretch your arms above your head, it works your body from head to toe, enhancing the strength of your foot, leg, arm and shoulder muscles, and mobilizing your shoulder joints. Your spine is stretched and, while you are moving steadily and breathing rhythmically, you deepen your breath and balance with each inhalation and exhalation.

Balance is also necessary for maintaining this asana: You must constantly stabilize your stance through very small movements of your foot and leg muscles.

Be gentle with your knees by keeping them aligned with your ankles, and be gentle with your arms and shoulders by positioning them in a way that is comfortable for you.

Start at a moderate pace, increasing it as you gradually gain strength.

If you continue from the eye exercises, first get into the squat position and slowly rise into the standing mountain posture.

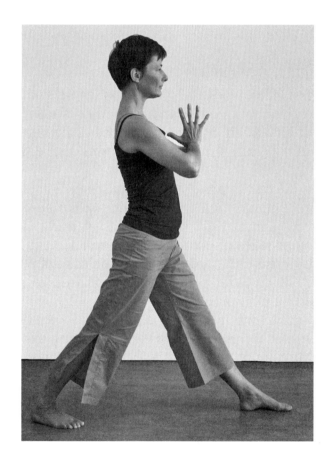

Place your feet hip width apart, weight evenly distributed on your feet. Extend your knees (do not hyperextend them), rotate your thighs outward, and tighten your pelvic muscles. Stretch the vertebrae between your tailbone and the crown of your head, lower your chin toward your chest, relax your shoulders and arms as well as your face and tongue muscles.

Breathe in and out deeply through your nose.

Put your left foot forward. Make sure that your feet are still hip width apart, with the outer sides of your feet parallel to one another, and your weight evenly distributed on both feet. Keep both legs stretched and both heels on the floor.

Push palms together in front of your sternum.

Inhale while slowly bending your front knee, and raising and opening your arms. Align your front knee over your ankle, tighten your pelvic muscles, and stretch your spine. Turn your face upward.

Exhale while slowly moving back into the starting position, consciously pushing your hands together again and stretching your front knee.

Repeat the exercise for six full inhalations and exhalations.

As you inhale, bring your right foot forward to return to the starting position.

Close your eyes and compare the feeling in both legs, both sides of your pelvis, and both sides of your face.

Open your eyes and repeat the exercise on the other side, putting your right foot forward this time.

Finally, get into the mountain posture, close your eyes, and compare both sides again. Feel the stretch of your back and the balancing effect of the whole exercise.

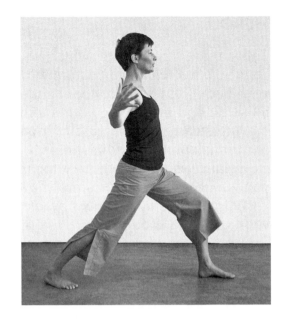

Reference Posture

The hero 1 posture gives your whole body a complete stretch from head to toe. Because widening the chest and deepening the breath is most important for women after surgery, the modified posture should be a regular part of your yoga practice—even after you are able to fully stretch out both arms above your head.

Come into the standing posture.

Put your left foot forward. Make sure that your feet are still hip width apart and that the outer sides of your feet are parallel. Keep both legs stretched and both heels on the floor.

Bring your palms together in front of your sternum.

As you inhale bend your left knee while stretching out your arms and looking upward. Make sure your front knee is properly aligned over your ankle.

Hold this posture for six full inhalations and exhalations.

Exhale and slowly move back into the standing posture. Close your eyes and compare both sides: both legs, both sides of your pelvis, both arms, and both sides of your face.

Repeat the exercise on the right side.

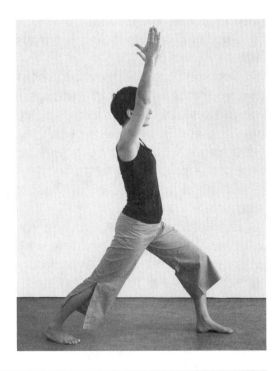

KNEE ROTATIONS

This is the same exercise we showed lying on the back in the chapter 2, but now you do it standing. Try it both ways and compare. The two variations are meant to align the bones and ligaments of your knee joints.

Knee problems are quite common and often hinder exercising. Standing and seated postures are good ways to get started if you are not comfortable with the standing versions. The following rotations of your knees will help you find the proper alignment.

For women undergoing cancer treatment, pain in the joints is often a side effect of the hormonal treatment. Pain in the knees can also be caused by sudden side-to-side movements, long hours of sitting with your knees bent, blockage in the knees from standing, or from having your knees extended while lying in bed. Knee problems are often accompanied by poor positioning of the torso: weak thigh muscles fail to keep the pelvis aligned and put excess weight on the knees.

Continue from the modified hero 1 posture or move into the standing posture.

Bend both your knees, and put your hands on top of your kneecaps, with your fingers facing inward.

Stretch your spine fully, and do not bow your head.

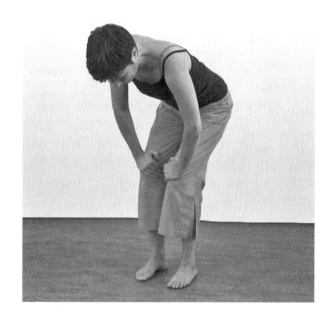

Slowly rotate your knees in one direction while maintaining a regular rhythm of movement and breathing. Become aware of blockages and noises in your joints.

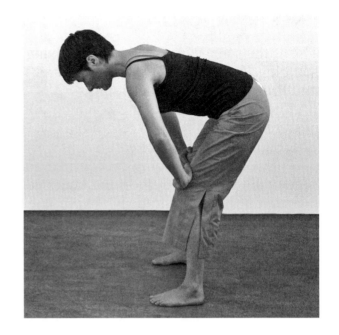

After a while change direction and do the rotation to the other side. Once again, pay attention to any blockages and noises.

Gently stop the movement, roll your body upward with your knees bent, and move into the standing posture. Feel the effects in your knees. Close your eyes if you like.

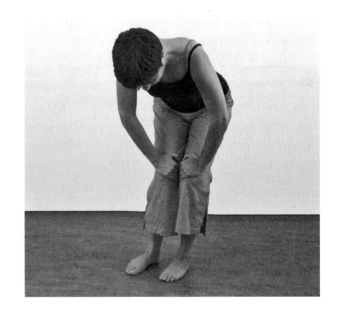

STARGAZER

Like the modified hero 1 posture, the stargazer posture allows you to widen your chest, mobilize your shoulder joints, stretch and gently bend your spine, and deepen your breath. The tightening of the pelvic muscles prevents pain in the lower back.

Continue from the knee rotation, or move into the standing posture.

Put your right foot forward, making sure that your feet are hip width apart and that the outer sides of your feet are parallel to one another. Distribute your weight evenly on your feet, keeping both legs stretched and your heels on the floor.

Bring both forearms behind your back and cross them.

As you inhale, stretch your spinal column and look upward. Make sure your pelvic muscles are tight.

Maintain the position for six full inhalations and exhalations.

As you inhale, bring your left foot forward, and return to the starting position.

Close your eyes and compare the feeling in both your legs, both sides of your pelvis, both shoulders, and both sides of your face.

Repeat the exercise on the other side, stepping forward with your left foot.

Bring both forearms behind your back. Cross your forearms so that the arm that was on the bottom in the first part of the exercise is now on top. (If it feels strange, you're doing it correctly. We all tend to put the same arm [hand, finger, etc.] on top if we bring both sides unconsciously together.)

Maintain the position for six full inhalations and exhalations.

Finally, get into the standing posture, close your eyes, and feel the effects of the whole exercise.

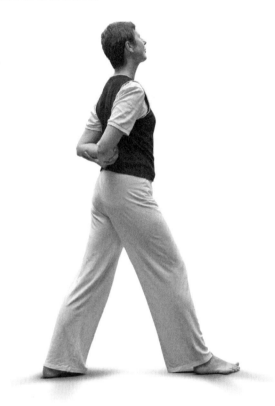

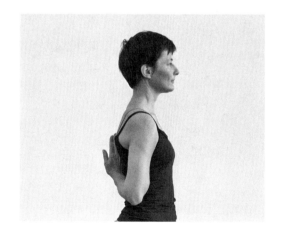

Reference Posture

The reference version of the stargazer posture looks impressive. Both versions serve to the same purpose: they widen the chest and mobilize the shoulder joints.

HIP ROTATIONS

This well known and simple exercise mobilizes foot, knee and hip joints, and makes you feel good.

Place both feet on the ground and move your pelvis slowly.

Continue from the modified star gazer posture or move into the standing posture.

Place your feet wider than hip width apart, with the outer sides of your feet parallel to one another, and your weight evenly distributed on your feet.

Extend your knees, making sure not to hyperextend them.

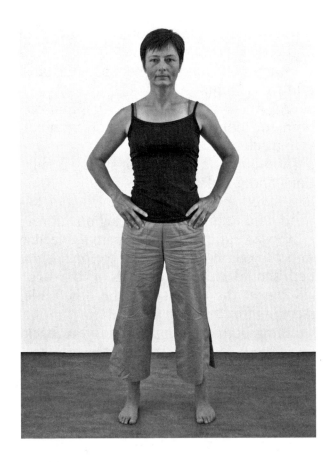

You can either place your hands on your hips or let your arms hang loosely to your sides.

Start moving your pelvis slowly in a circle, and keep to a steady breathing rhythm. Expand the movement.

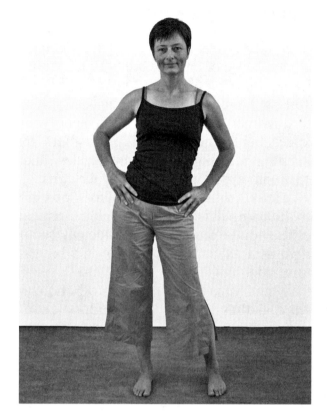

After a while, change the direction of the hip rotation and continue the exercise.

Finally, stop the rotation and return into the standing posture. Feel the effects of the steady rotation.

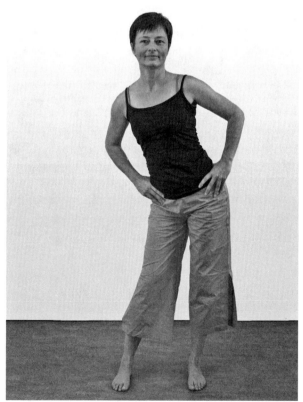

HERO 2

Strength in your foot and leg muscles and a good sense of balance are both necessary for maintaining the hero 2 posture because you have to constantly stabilize your stance through very small movements. Keep your knees bent, and be gentle with them by keeping them aligned with your ankles. Take care with the proper height of your arms.

Hero 2 differs from the hero 1 posture in that the pelvis is open to the side instead of the front. Your pelvis is in line with your right and left legs, depending on which is forward.

Many yoga students tend to bend forward as they lift their arms and look over their leading arm. To prevent this, stretch your spine and keep your torso centered. Pay attention to your arms and shoulders and keep them in a position that works comfortably with your actual fitness level. Start moderately and gradually increase your pace.

> *"I love both hero postures. In hero 1, you open your arms, but in hero 2 you raise your arms and strengthen your legs at the same time."*

> *"I liked the hero posture 2 because I could look over my stretched-out arm and feel the energy in my body."*

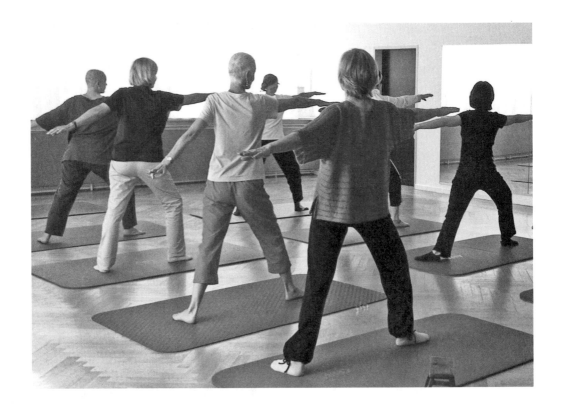

Continue from the hip rotation, or move into the standing posture. Move your feet to the sides, one leg length apart.

Turn your left foot completely outward, and turn your right foot 45 degrees inward.

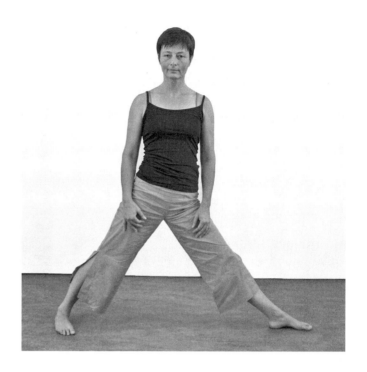

Exhale and slowly bend your left knee forward until it is above your ankle. Your right leg is stretched.

Inhale while slowly raising your arms up to shoulder height. Stretch out both arms. If you are straining, lower or bend one arm.

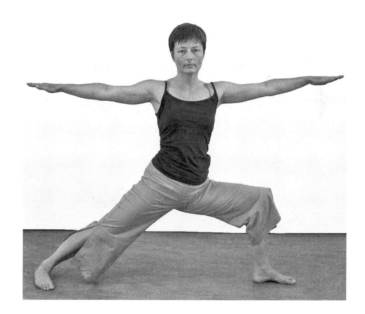

Stretch your spine again, turn your head, and look over your left arm. Make sure that your torso is in an upright position.

Maintain the position for six full inhalations and exhalations.

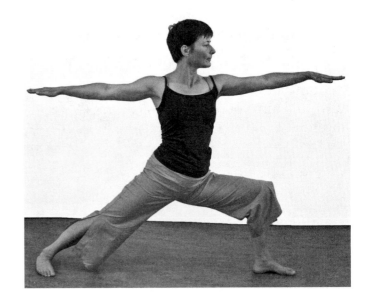

As you inhale, stretch both legs and lower your arms.

Bring your feet together until they are hip width apart and compare the sides of your body: both legs, both sides of your pelvis, both shoulders, and both sides of your face.

Repeat the posture on the right side.

Finally, return to the standing posture and feel the energy in your body. Close your eyes if you like.

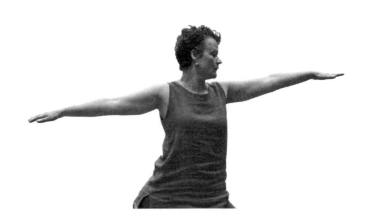

Variation

If one arm cannot be fully stretched out, bend your arm to your comfort when you are beginning to exercise.

PYRAMID

The modified pyramid posture stretches your legs and spine in a forward bend. To be gentle with your lower back, consciously stretch your spine and look downward to stay aligned. Keep your knees moderately bent, and your pelvis muscles tightened throughout the whole exercise.

Continue from the hero 2 posture, or move into the standing posture.

Position your feet one leg length apart, with the outer sides of both feet touching the floor. Bend your knees.
Inhale and stretch out your spine.
Exhale while slowly bending down until your torso is parallel to the floor.

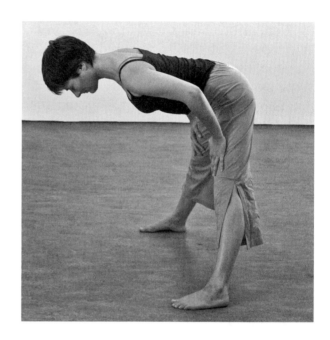

Lower your arms until your fingers or hands touch the floor. Make sure that your wrists are under your shoulder joints.

With the next exhalation slowly bend your right knee. Make sure that the outer sides of your feet are still on the floor.

Inhale while slowly moving back into the middle.

Exhale while slowly bending your left knee.

Inhale while slowly moving back into the middle.

Repeat the bends and stretches for six complete inhalations and exhalations.

Stop the movement, and stretch your spine again.

As you inhale, slowly roll your torso upward.

Bring your feet closer together, and move into the standing posture. Feel the effects of the exercise. Close your eyes if you like.

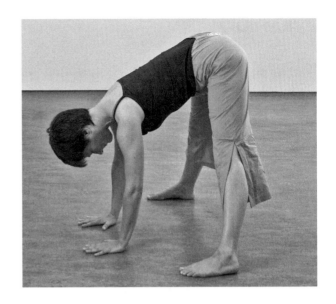

Variations

If your fingers cannot touch the ground, use a folded blanket, a big book, or blocks (most yoga schools have them) to place your hands on. Be sure you stretch your back and do not bend your spine to reach the floor.

TREE POSTURE

Both the tree posture and the knee rotation posture are done twice during the yoga class: at the beginning in a supine posture, and at the end of the dynamic section in a standing position.

In an upright position, this posture enhances the strength of your foot, leg, and arm muscles and challenges your sense of balance.

To allow maximum levels of concentration and safety, this posture is shown at a beginner's level. If you feel safe after practicing for a while, close your eyes during the asana.

Continue from the modified pyramid posture, or move into the standing posture.

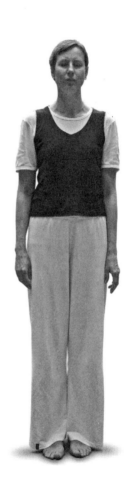

Push your palms together in front of your sternum. Relax your shoulders, facial muscles, lips, and tongue.

Shift your weight to your right leg.

While inhaling, bend your left leg and push the sole of your left foot against the inner side of your inner right ankle. Rotate your bent leg outward as far as possible.

Maintain this posture for six complete inhalations and exhalations.

As you exhale, slowly turn your left leg back to the middle, stretch it out, and place it hip width apart from your right foot.

Close your eyes and compare both sides of your body: left and right leg, left and right sides of your pelvis, and left and right sides of your face.

Repeat the exercise on the other side.

Finally, return to the standing posture and again feel both sides of your body. Close your eyes if you like.

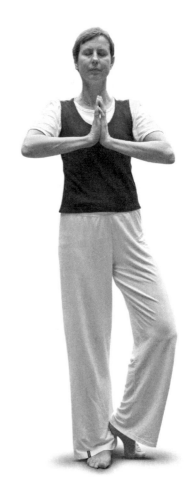

Reference Posture

These postures are more challenging in terms of balance. If you have a good sense of balance and have tried the modified version, try the tree posture with your foot against the inner side of your knee instead of your ankle.

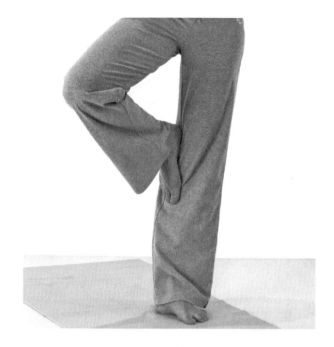

Alternatively, you can also place the sole of your foot against your inner thigh.

In all cases, make sure that your bent knee is rotated to the outside and that your pelvis is erect.

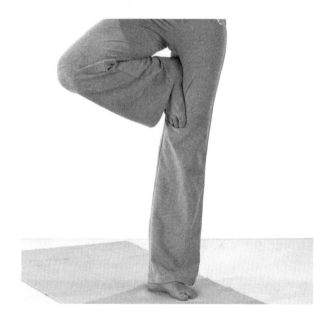

TRIANGLE IN MOTION

After practicing back and forward bends, rotations, and balancing postures, we continue the dynamic section with a side bend. Make sure that you are actually bending to the side and feeling the stretch in your flanks. Be gentle with your body. If you have difficulties fully stretching both sides, start with one side and bend the arm of the side that is weaker. Take your time feeling the effects of the exercise, and slowly move on to more challenging versions of the posture.

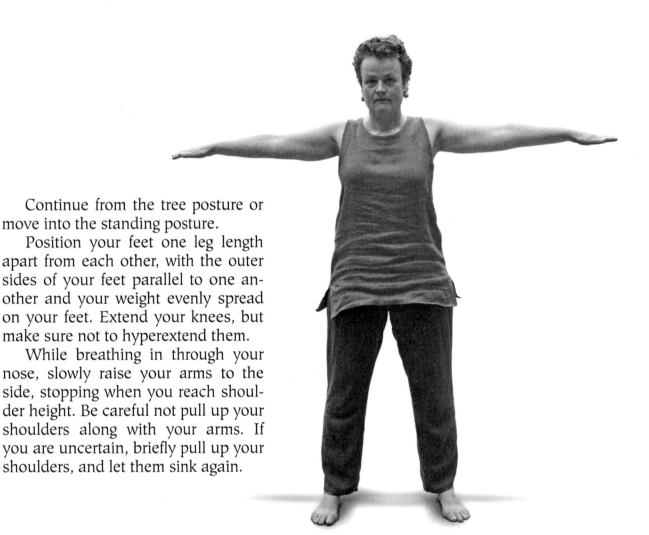

Continue from the tree posture or move into the standing posture.

Position your feet one leg length apart from each other, with the outer sides of your feet parallel to one another and your weight evenly spread on your feet. Extend your knees, but make sure not to hyperextend them.

While breathing in through your nose, slowly raise your arms to the side, stopping when you reach shoulder height. Be careful not pull up your shoulders along with your arms. If you are uncertain, briefly pull up your shoulders, and let them sink again.

Exhale and slowly bend your torso to the left while your left arm is moving downward and your right arm is moving upward. (You do not actually move your arms, they move with your torso.) Do this cautiously, and check whether or not the upper arm feels good. If it doesn't, either lower your arm or bend it. Feel the stretch in your right flank.

Inhale and return into the starting position.

Exhale and slowly bend your torso to the right while your left arm is moving upward, and your right arm is moving downward. Check again whether the upper arm feels good, and, if not, either lower your arm or bend it. Feel the stretch in your left flank.

Repeat the whole exercise for six full inhalations and exhalations.

After the sixth turn, keep the posture for three full breathing cycles on each side.

Return into the standing position with an inhalation.

Exhale and lower your arms.

Finally, remain in the standing posture and feel the stretch of your flanks. Close your eyes if you like.

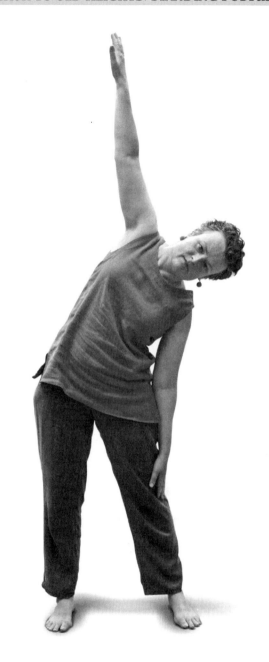

Variation

Start with gentle movements. If your upper arm does not feel good, lower or bend it.

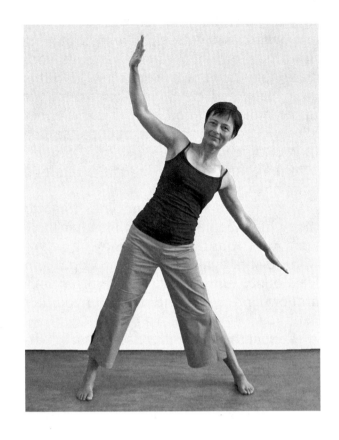

Reference Posture

In the triangle posture, you get the maximum stretch of your flanks as you hold the posture for six breathing cycles.

Come into the standing posture. Turn your left foot outward with the toes pointing forward, and turn your right foot inward 45 degrees.

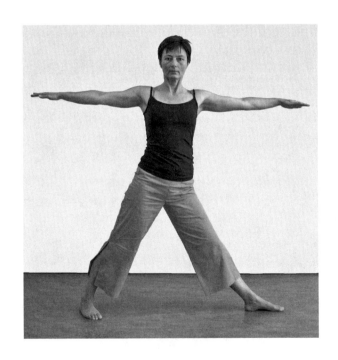

Inhale while raising your arms until they are fully stretched out at shoulder height. Make sure that you did not pull up your shoulders. If you are uncertain, you can briefly raise your shoulders and let them sink again.

Exhale while bending your torso to the left side. Both arms are stretched.

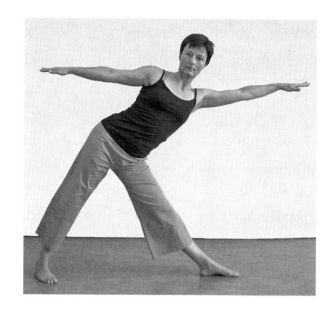

Continue the movement, pointing your left arm downward and your right arm upward. Make sure you do not bend your torso forward. Keep both your flanks stretched and keep your head and neck straight. Maintain the posture for six complete inhalations and exhalations.

As you inhale, return to the upright position, and place your feet hip width apart. Compare both sides of your body: your legs, both sides of your pelvis, both sides of your shoulders, and your face.

Repeat the posture on the other side.

Finally, with an inhalation, return to the upright position, and place both your feet hip width apart. Feel the effects of the stretches in your flanks. Close your eyes if you like.

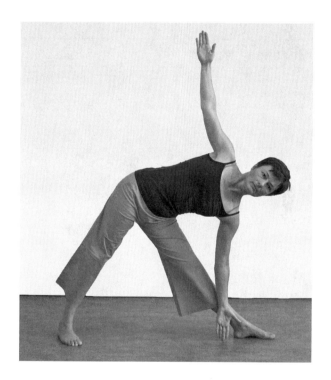

QUICK LOOK

Chapter 11 BACK TO OLD HEIGHTS: STANDING POSTURES	
Hero 1	Enhances the strength of foot, leg, and arm muscles; mobilizes the shoulder joints; and widens the chest.
Knee Rotations	Aligns the bones and ligaments of the knee joints.
Stargazer	Widens the chest, mobilizes the shoulder joints, stretches the spine, and deepens the breath.
Hip Rotations	Mobilizes foot, knee and hip joints.
Hero 2	Develops the strength of foot, leg, and arm muscles and increases the sense of balance.
Pyramid	Stretches legs and spine in a forward bend.
Tree Posture	Enhances the strength of foot, leg, and arm muscles and challenges the sense of balance in an upright position.
Triangle in Motion	Provides a stretch for your flanks.

Once Again:
Postures for Neck,
Shoulders, and Arms

Because it is vital to exercise hands, arms, and shoulders, we do these postures twice during the yoga class: in a supine posture at the beginning of the class and then seated or standing after the dynamic section. Compare the effects of the exercises done lying on the back with those done seated or standing. The following exercises can and should be done several times during the day, so we'll present more of them to you in part III: Yoga for Moments in Between.

Nerve injury to the shoulder and back muscles can occur after the removal of lymph nodes from the armpit and, unfortunately, lymphedema can develop. Lymph vessels help transport tissue fluid back into circulation with the blood; and the removal of the lymph nodes disrupts this process and can lead to the accumulation of fluid and swelling of the hands or arms. The risk of developing lymphedema increases after radiation therapy. For a short time, wearing surgical hose can help, but, in the long run, it is vital to exercise and manually perform lymph drainage.

The arm and shoulder exercises in this section will help you avoid developing or aggravating lymphedema.

Besides doing these postures regularly during the day and in your yoga class, we recommend the following:

Do not carry heavy objects with your affected arm.

Avoid long sunbaths and visits to the sauna.

Make sure to use your healthy arm when taking your blood pressure or providing a blood sample.

Take all precautions necessary to avoid infection in the affected arm.

Sleep on your healthy side.

Make sure that you're able to perform manual lymph drainage; it's important in developing self-reliance.

ARM LIFTS

Because one unconsciously tries to reduce the movement of arms and shoulders after surgery, it is helpful to give them special attention. Following breast surgeries, it is vital to exercise hands, arms, and shoulders.

Continue from triangle in motion, or come into the standing posture.

Place your feet hip width apart, and distribute your weight evenly on your feet.

Extend your knees (but do not hyperextend them), and rotate your thighs outward.

Tighten your pelvic muscles, and stretch the vertebrae between your tailbone and the crown of your head.

Lower your chin toward your chest, and relax your shoulders and arms along with your face and tongue muscles.

Breathe in and out deeply through your nose.

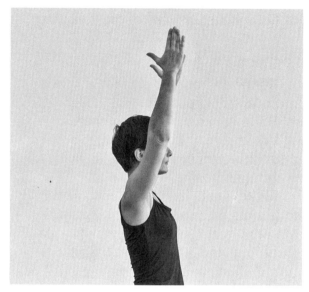

As you inhale, lift your arms upward toward the ceiling, making sure not to lift your shoulders. Stretch your arms as far as possible. Check if the stretch feels good, and, if not, reduce the stretch in one or both arms.

Open and close your hands (pumping).

Repeat the movement during six inhalations and exhalations.

As you exhale, lower your arms.

Feel the effect of the exercise. Close your eyes if you like.

ARM ROTATIONS

The arm rotation exercise counters the poor posture of shoulders that accompanies shallow breathing. This one is especially effective at mobilizing the shoulder joints and strengthening the arm muscles. Exercises for neck, shoulder, and arm muscles can be done in all postures: lying, sitting, and standing. Here, we show you how to perform the rotations while standing.

Once again, a word of caution: Make sure not to overdo the exercise.

Continue from the arm lift or move into a standing posture.

Place your feet hip width apart.

While breathing in through your nose, slowly raise your arms sideways to shoulder height.

Make sure that you are raising your arms only, not your shoulders. If you are uncertain, briefly pull up your shoulders, and let them sink again.

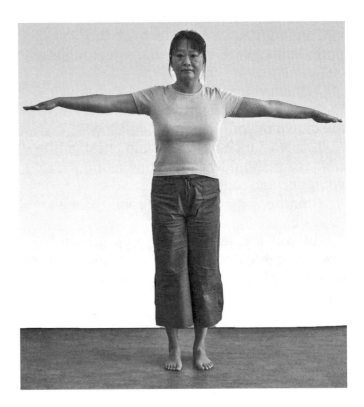

As you exhale, rotate your stretched arms backward until your palms are facing backward.

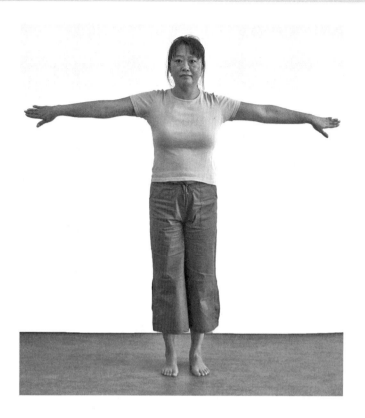

As you inhale, rotate your stretched arms forward until your palms are facing forward.

Repeat this rotation of your stretched arms for six complete breathing cycles.

Stop the movement. Inhale and stretch your arms again.

As you exhale, slowly lower your arms.

Return to the standing posture and feel the effects. Close your eyes if you like.

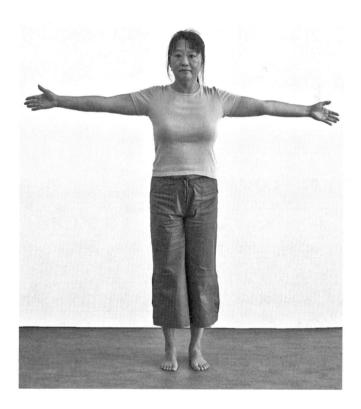

ARM BENDS

Here, we present another posture that gives special attention to your arms and shoulders by gently strengthening your muscles.

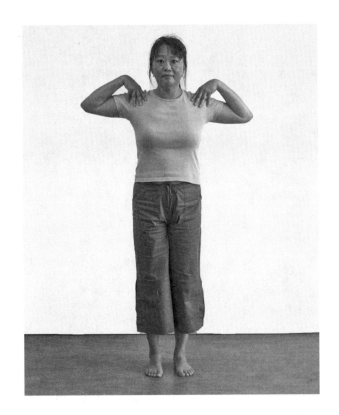

Continue from the arm rotation, or move into a seated, standing, or kneeling posture.

Place your feet hip width apart.

While breathing in through your nose, slowly raise your arms sideways to shoulder height. Make sure that you are raising your arms only, not your shoulders. If you are uncertain, briefly pull up your shoulders, and let them sink again.

As you exhale, bend both arms up so your hands touch the tops of your shoulders.

As you inhale, stretch both arms again.

Repeat the movements for six complete breathing cycles.

Stop the movement. Inhale and stretch your arms again.

As you exhale, slowly lower your arms.

Return to the standing posture, and feel the effects. Close your eyes if you like.

QUICK LOOK

Chapter 12 ONCE AGAIN: POSTURES FOR NECK, SHOULDERS, AND ARMS	
Arm Lifts	Exercises hands, arms, and shoulders, and supports the transport of tissue fluid back into the circulation.
Arm Rotations	Mobilizes the shoulder joints and strengthens the arm muscles.
Arm Bends	Supports the transport of tissue fluid back into the circulation and exercises arm muscles

Back to the Mat:
More Supine Postures

After the dynamic part of the yoga lesson, we return to the floor with another set of supine postures. These postures particularly support stretching and muscle building, especially of the abdominal muscles. When you lack full strength in your arms, belly muscles are important because they can help you pull yourself up out of bed, for example. Because belly muscles function in perfect opposition to the back muscles, we train both sets in the next section. We start with the boat posture to strengthen the belly muscles, continue with the shoulder bridge to enhance the flexibility and strength of the back and leg muscles, and do a variation of the already introduced knee-to-chest exercise as a balancing posture. We then do a set of stretches and counter stretches, performed in a safe supine posture. Alignments are addressed in the detailed description of each asana.

BOAT POSTURE

Continue from the arm bend exercise, or move into the seated posture on the floor. Bend your knees, position your feet on the floor, and distribute your weight evenly on both sit bones. Place your hands around your knees.

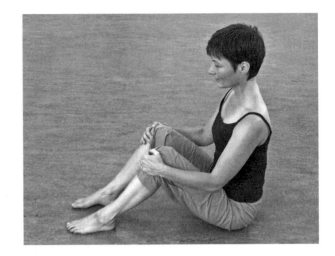

Keep your pelvis in an upright position and stretch your entire spinal column. Extend the crown of your head upward, raise your sternum, and relax your face and mouth muscles. Breathe in and out deeply through your nose.

While you inhale, stretch your arms forward. Maintain the posture during six complete inhalations and exhalations.

Get back into the starting posture and feel the effects. Close your eyes if you like.

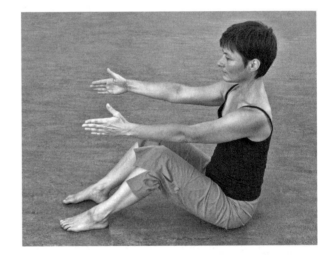

Boat Posture in Motion

To build up your belly muscles, you can vary the posture and move your torso back and forth.

As you inhale, move your torso backward.
As you exhale, move your torso forward, and come back into the starting position.
Begin with small movements, and keep your spine stretched out.
Repeat the movement during six complete inhalations and exhalations.

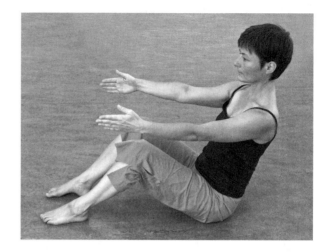

Reference Posture

If you want to exercise the full posture, make sure that you have enough space behind you to completely lay down. Come into the starting position, place your hands around your knees, and stretch your spine and your arms. As you inhale, move your torso backward, placing your back on the floor, vertebra by vertebra. Keep your arms stretched out as you move. As you exhale, return to the starting position.

SHOULDER BRIDGE

The shoulder bridge, performed immediately after the boat posture, enhances the strength and flexibility of the back and leg muscles. Though it is a backward bend, it is safely supported by your feet, arms, shoulders, and head.

As you lift your body, make sure that you bend and stretch your spine vertebra by vertebra.

Check that you are correctly aligned. Place your feet hip width apart, keep your knees parallel, tighten your pelvic muscles, stretch your neck, and point your chin toward your chest. Before continuing, make sure your arms can carry the weight. Start by raising only the lower part of your spine, and, if it feels good, continue up to your shoulder blades.

Part I

If you continue from the boat posture, place your hands on both sides of your hips. As you inhale, move your torso backward, and place your back on the floor vertebra by vertebra. If you are practicing on a mat, move upward to use the whole length of your mat.

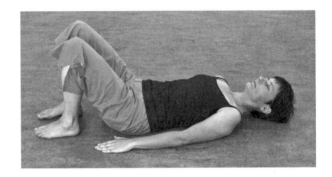

Bend both your legs, and place your feet hip width apart on the floor.

Place your arms on the floor by your sides, palms facing downward.

Inhale through your nose, and tighten your pelvic muscles as you lift your back vertebra by vertebra, starting with the tailbone.

Exhale through your nose while lowering your back vertebra by vertebra. Relax your pelvis muscles at the end of the movement.

Make sure your breathing and movement are completely synchronized.

Repeat the movements for six complete inhalations and exhalations.

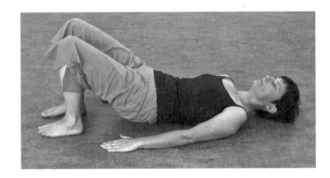

Part II

To do the complete asana, inhale through your nose and tighten your bottom (pelvic muscles) while lifting your back vertebra by vertebra. Make sure your feet push into the floor.

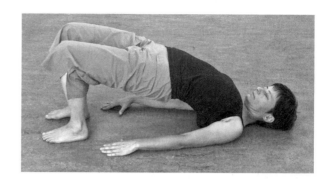

Maintain the posture for six complete inhalations and exhalations.

Exhale as you lower your spine vertebra by vertebra, and return the starting position.

Stretch out your legs and feel the effects of the back bend. Close your eyes if it feels comfortable.

KNEES TO CHEST

If you continue from the shoulder bridge posture (a backward bend), the knee to chest posture serves as a balancing posture. The lower part of your spine bends up during this exercise.

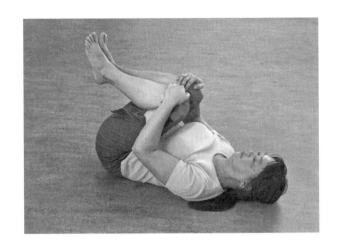

Proceed from the shoulder bridge, or begin by lying on your back.

Consciously stretch your spine. Stretch your neck, lower your chin toward your sternum, and relax your face, lips, and tongue.

Bend your knees, and pull them to your chest.

Place your right hand on your right knee and your left hand on your left knee. Relax your lower legs and feet, and stretch your neck.

Exhale through your nose, bend your arms, and pull your knees closer to your chest.

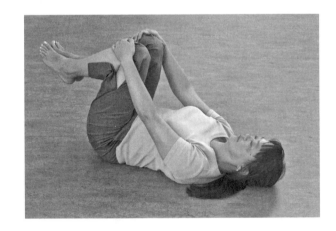

Inhale through your nose, stretch your arms, and move your knees away from your chest.

Repeat the movement during at least six complete inhalations and exhalations.

Place your feet back on the floor, and feel the effects of the movement. Close your eyes if you like.

Variation

Instead of moving back and forth, you can move in circles.

Begin with small clockwise circles and expand them.

Do the same in the opposite direction.

Exhale while you do the lower half of the circle, and inhale while you do the upper half.

Feel how your lower back is massaged.

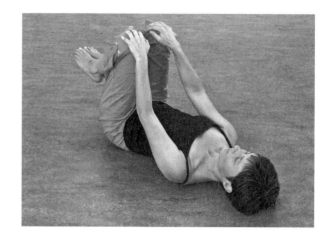

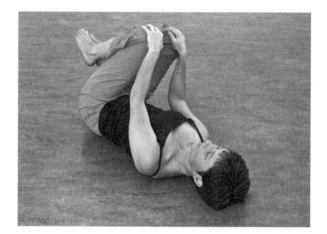

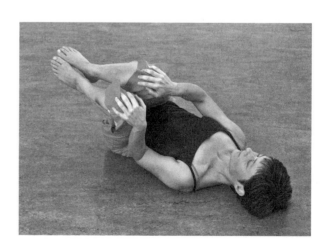

QUICK LOOK

Chapter 13 BACK TO THE MAT: MORE SUPINE POSTURES	
Boat Posture	Develops the strength of your belly and back muscles.
Shoulder Bridge	Enhance the flexibility and strength of the back and leg muscles.
Knees to Chest	A gentle, forward bend of the lower spine that also serves as a balancing posture.

Time to Feel the Effects: Relaxing Postures

In yoga, it is important to exercise regularly, and to ascertain what is best for you in specific situations. The more often you have been in a posture, the better you are able to evaluate your body tone, breathing rhythm, and depth of breathing, and the more aware you will become of your thoughts and feelings. A lot of women in our study enjoyed all kinds of sports, and they often told us what a difference yoga made to their experience doing athletics, especially in terms of breathing and awareness.

The two following yoga postures enable you to become aware of the effects of the yoga class and of the difference in your body tone, feelings, and thoughts while doing the same exercises in various settings and at different times during the day.

Remember to stretch your neck, and lift your head a little to prevent any bowing while turning it.

"You always told us: 'Recognize your thoughts and feelings.' I'm not a person with high self-awareness. I love jogging and ball games. But I must admit, yoga helped me feel good."

KAYA KRIYA

Kaya kriya develops your ability to simultaneously breathe and move, focuses your attention, and provides gentle training for the joints.

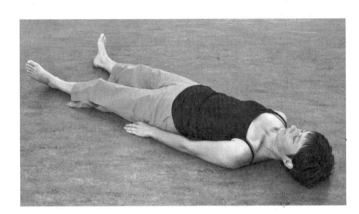

Continue from the knee to chest posture, or lie on your back.

Stretch your entire spine.

Stretch your neck, and lower your chin toward your sternum.

Close your eyes.

Relax your face and the muscles of your mouth.

Relax your shoulders so that they lie flat on the floor.

Lay your arms beside your body, palms facing the floor.

Place your legs several inches apart, leaving enough space between your feet for your big toes to touch when you rotate your feet.

Rotate your feet outward.

Breathe in and out deeply through your nose.

Place your arms very close to your sides.

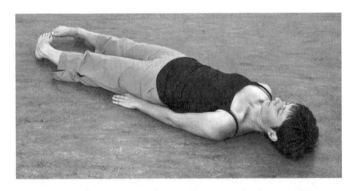

As you inhale, rotate your feet inward until your big toes touch.

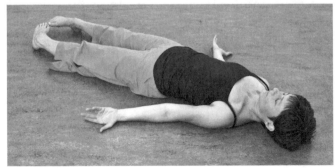

Rotate your arms outward away from your sides.

Turn your head to the right (without bowing your head).

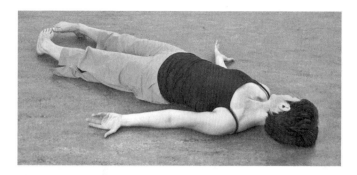

As you exhale, rotate your feet outward.

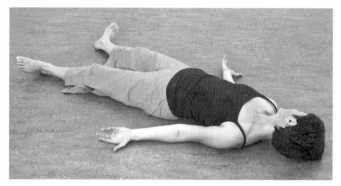

Rotate your arms toward your sides.

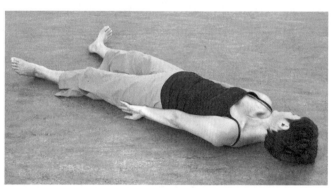

Turn your head to the left.

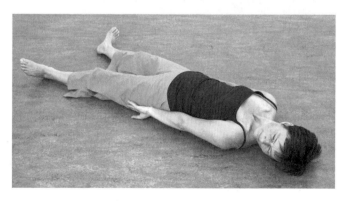

Repeat the movements for six complete inhalations and exhalations.

Return to the starting position, with your arms, palms up, by your sides, and feet rotated outward. Feel the effects of kaya kriya.

YOGA NIDRA

Yoga nidra is one of the best ways to become aware of the effects yoga has on different parts of your body. The first step is to lie down in shanti asana, and become aware of your body part by part.

You can either develop your own way of moving your awareness through your body or be guided by a teacher (either in a class or at home using a CD). Both methods have their advantages.

Practicing on your own can be helpful if you have trouble falling asleep, but requires regular practice and the development of a rhythm as you move your attention from body part to body part.

Bringing the awareness toward a certain part of the body while listening to a voice is very relaxing, and doing yoga nidra this way can give you the feeling of being directly connected to your body without using words, terms, or images.

There is generally no correct way of doing yoga nidra, just find a way that works best for you as an individual.

> *"Sometimes when I am absentminded—and it is not owing to my illness—I like to stretch out on the floor and become aware of my body in yoga nidra."*

Continue from kaya krya, or start in shanti asana.

Bring your attention to your left foot, your left sole, your left ankle, your left lower leg, your left knee, your left thigh, your left hip joint.

Bring your attention to your right foot, your right sole, your right ankle, your right lower leg, your right knee, your right thigh, your right hip joint.

Bring your attention to your left hand, your left palm, your left wrist, your left lower arm, your left elbow, your left upper arm, your left shoulder joint.

Bring your attention to your right hand, your right palm, your right wrist, your right lower arm, your right elbow, your right upper arm, your right shoulder joint.

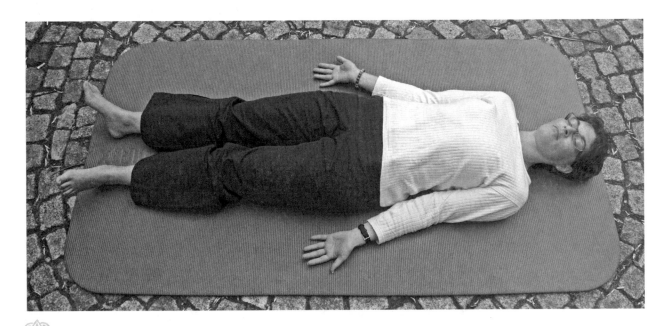

Bring your attention to the back of your head where it lies on the floor, to the front of your face, your right brow, your left brow, your right eye, your left eye, the tip of your nose, your upper lip, your lower lip, the tip of your chin.

Bring your attention to your belly, observe how it moves up and down. Keep your attention on your belly for a couple of inhalations and exhalations.

To get out of the posture, inhale and exhale completely through your nose a couple of times.

Make small movements with your toes and fingers, with your feet and hands, your legs and arms. Stretch your body if it feels good.

Get up into a seated posture.

In an upright posture on the floor, feel the effects of yoga nidra with your eyes closed.

QUICK LOOK

Chapter 14 TIME TO FEEL THE EFFECTS: RELAXING POSTURES	
Kaya Kriya	Helps you simultaneously breathe and move, focuses the attention, and is also a gentle exercise for the joints.
Yoga Nidra	One of the best ways to recognize the effects yoga has on different parts of the body.

Round Out
Your Practice:
Energizing Postures

The full yoga class we offered during our study ended with energizing postures. Done in an upright seated position, these relaxing postures provide a time at the end of the class to feel the difference in your body tone, awareness, and thoughts from the beginning of the class.

There are no contraindications for these postures. Make sure that you use caution when standing at the end of your yoga lesson; suddenly rising from calm stances can lead to a decrease in blood pressure and make you feel dizzy. Inhale while rolling upward into a standing position.

IMAGINATION

Earlier, we talked about the importance of exercising your arms and shoulders after surgery. Here, we present a yoga posture in which you will feel your arms in such a way that, without moving them, you get a sense of the flowing motion in your blood vessels. If you like this exercise, it can accompany your physical workout of arms and shoulders.

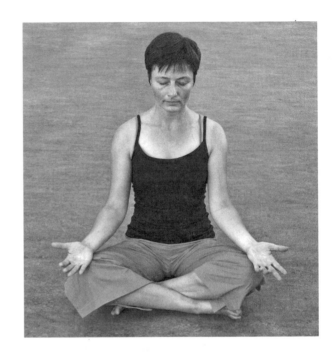

Continue from yoga nidra, or come into an upright seated posture. You may choose to sit with your legs crossed, to kneel, or to sit on a chair.

Place both hands on your knees, with the palms facing up toward the ceiling. Close your eyes. As you do this exercise, imagine energy moving up and down your arms. For women suffering from lymphedema, this exercise may be particularly helpful in imagining the renewed flow of blocked fluids.

Focus your attention on your left hand. Inhale through your nose, and move your attention up your left arm. Exhale through your nose, and move your attention to your right arm, then down to your hand.

Inhale through your nose, and move your attention up your right arm. Exhale through your nose, and move your attention down your left arm to your hand.

Repeat the exercise for six complete inhalations and exhalations.

Feel the effect of the posture in your starting position. Close your eyes if you like.

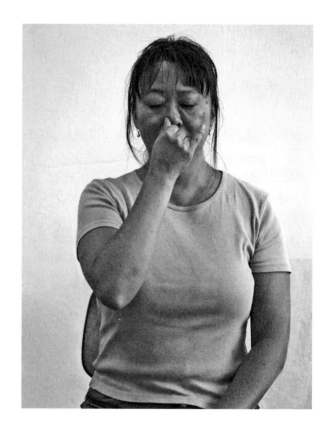

ALTERNATE NOSTRIL BREATHING

If your scars itch, or if you have an allergic reaction, you might unconsciously begin to take more shallow breaths. With the following yoga exercise, you can slowly develop a steady breathing rhythm, composed of a regular rhythm and complete inhalations and exhalations, while enhancing your ability to concentrate. Alternate nostril breathing, when practiced regularly, will allow you to determine if there are differences between your inhalations and exhalations. For some, it is easy to fully inhale but difficult to completely exhale, while for others it's the other way around.

> *"I felt handicapped and made small movements. And after a while I felt small. With yoga, I learned to completely inhale and exhale, widen my chest, and fully use my joints. Yoga helped me to open myself, stand up, and recognize my abilities."*

Continue from the imagination exercise, or come into a seated posture on the floor or on a chair.

Bend the index finger, middle finger, and ring finger of one hand, and stretch out your thumb and little finger.

Place your thumb next to your right nostril and your little finger next to the left nostril. Either place your bent arm on the table, or hold it comfortably in front of your body in such a way that it is not pushing on your thorax and does not block your breathing.

To begin, first breathe out deeply through both nostrils.

Then, close your right nostril with your thumb, and slowly breathe in through your left nostril. Maintain the position and feel your filled lungs.

Close the left nostril with your little finger, and slowly breathe out completely through the right nostril. Maintain the position and feel your "empty" lungs.

Slowly breathe in again through the same right nostril. Maintain the position, and feel your filled lungs. Close your right nostril with your thumb, and slowly breathe out through the left nostril again. Maintain the position and feel your "empty" lungs.

Repeat the alternate nostril breathing for at least six complete breath cycles.

Finally, lower your hand and breathe in and out through both your nostrils. Feel the calming effects. Keep your eyes closed if you like.

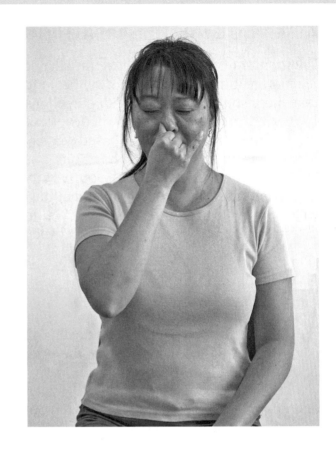

Variation

To achieve as even a breathing rhythm as possible, count to six between every inhalation and every exhalation and to three during the breaks in between. The volume of breath you take in and breathe out can be increased with time. After doing this exercise for a while, you can perform the exercises at a ratio of 8:4, 10:5, and more. This depends, however, on your ability to achieve a pleasant, thorough, and even breathing rhythm.

CHANTING

Chanting improves your regular breathing, helps you to gain a higher level of attentiveness, and increases self-esteem. If you practice the following little exercise regularly, your voice can also give you an idea of your actual fitness and energy.

Continue from alternate nostril breathing, or come into a seated posture on the floor or on a chair.

Place your hands on your thighs, palms facing downward.

Inhale through your nose, and exhale with the sound "aah."

Inhale through your nose, and exhale with the sound "ooh."

Inhale through your nose, and exhale with the sound "mmm."

Repeat each sound three times.

At the end of the chanting, note your thoughts and feelings.

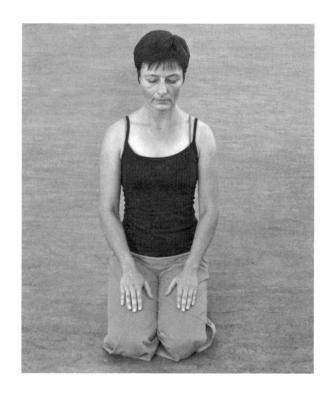

SEATED SHANTI ASANA

At the end of your practice, place your right hand into left hand (whether you are sitting or kneeling), a well-known gesture of concentration in yoga.

Keep the posture for a while before you open your eyes. Become aware of the changes in energy, strength, and flexibility after practicing.

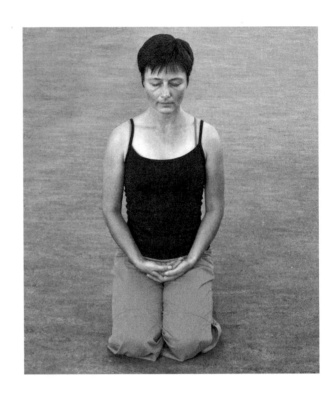

QUICK LOOK

Chapter 15 ROUND OUT YOUR PRACTICE: ENERGIZING POSTURES	
Imagination	Develops the awareness of arms and flowing motion in the blood vessels.
	Can accompany physical workout of arms and shoulders.
Alternate Nostril Breathing	Enhances breathing capacity and develops the ability to focus.
Chanting	Chanting is good for a regular breath, a better level of attentiveness, and greater self-esteem.
Seated Shanti Asana	Helps you concentrate and become aware of the effects after practicing yoga.

PART
III

YOGA POSTURES

FOR MOMENTS

IN BETWEEN

The yoga postures, or asanas, we show you in this third part, "Yoga for Moments in Between," are designed to provide immediate relief. They can be practiced at any time and in (almost) any place, and can relieve pain in the shoulders and arms, stretch your whole body, or relax and calm you. Each of them focuses on the part of the body mentioned. Luckily, most of the asanas also affect the body and mind in multiple ways; for example, standing positions for your back and shoulders also affect the legs, feet, and toes, and eye exercises also help calm the mind. Together with synchronized breathing, and with regular practice, these asanas have an immediate, positive effect. Develop your daily yoga practice by writing down which yoga postures you enjoy doing, and which postures have an immediate effect.

"You have told us to practice yoga 'in between.' While I do the washing, I place my feet and distribute my weight evenly. I rotate my thighs, tighten my pelvic muscles, and stretch my spine and my neck, up to the crown of my head. I also do this as soon as I feel my back starting to hurt. That relieves the whole thing."

Controlled relaxation is the key to physical and mental relief. By intentionally relaxing those muscles you are not using, you learn to more easily attain a relaxed posture in yoga as well as in everyday life. In addition, the more synchronized your breathing and movement, the more profound your musculoskeletal relaxation will be when you exhale, which will help you counteract chronic tension. Yoga also trains your brain to recognize varying stimulants and identify their locations and causes: a challenging stretch, a flowing movement, a relaxation that comes with exhalation, the composition of different body surfaces, as well as fine temperature differences. Practicing yoga eventually becomes as effective as receiving a good massage. Even those who had practiced on and off before found that regular practice changed the way they felt and helped them take themselves and their bodies seriously.

"After practicing yoga intensively for a year, I could consciously feel what it does to my body and mind. I learned yoga again in a new way. And my impression of yoga was now from the perspective of a sick person, focusing on how yoga could positively influence my body."

Stretch and Relax
Your Back

MOUNTAIN POSTURE

Yoga postures, such as the hero 2, immediately improve your sense of strength. The mountain postures serves the same purpose and can be done discreetly while you wait for an elevator or a green light, while you are on the phone, and so on.

The mountain posture is easy to do and very beneficial, especially if you feel small or hunched, because you stretch the whole body, maintain balance, and increase focus.

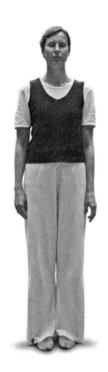

Place your feet hip width apart, and distribute your weight evenly on your feet. If you feel more weight on the inner side of your feet (or vice versa), adjust accordingly.

Extend your knees, making sure not to hyperextend them.

Rotate your thighs outward and feel your pelvis lifting up.

Support this position of your pelvis by tightening your pelvic muscles.

Stretch the vertebrae from your tailbone to the crown of your head.

Relax your belly.

Raise your sternum, and let your shoulders and arms hang down loosely.

Align your chin parallel to the ground, and relax your face, lips, and tongue.

Breathe in and out deeply through your nose.

Variation

You can stretch your spine while sitting on a chair or in a car.

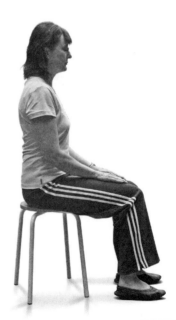

TURTLE POSTURE

The turtle posture is a forward bend, useful for when you feel the need to relax your shoulders or enlarge the space between your vertebrae. If you suffer from uncontrolled high blood pressure or from eye and ear conditions, do the tiger breathing posture instead.

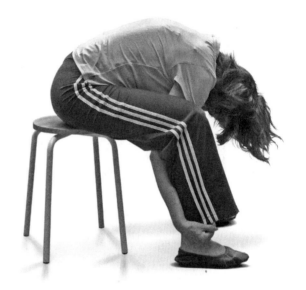

Sit down on a chair. Place your feet more than hip width apart from one another and place your knee joints above your ankles. Pull your pelvis upright, stretch your spine, extend the crown of your head upward, and lower your chin toward your sternum. Relax your shoulders and arms, as well as your face and tongue muscles.

Place your hands on top of your thighs.

Inhale through your nose while in this position.

Exhale and gently bend downward between your knees, placing your hands around your lower legs or ankles. Relax your neck muscles.

Maintain the position for three complete inhalations. With each exhalation, relax your shoulders. With each inhalation, feel the stretch of your spine.

As you inhale, stretch your spine and raise your stretched torso back into the starting position.

Keep your eyes closed, and feel the effect of the exercise.

Variation

You can bend forward and place your forearms on your knees. Rest your head on your upper arm.

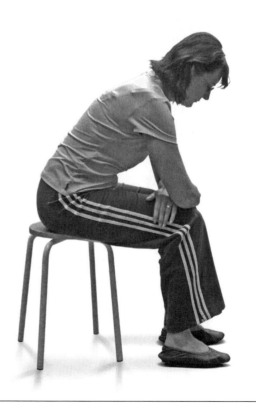

TIGER BREATHING

Like the turtle posture, tiger breathing enhances your awareness of your spine, releases the tension in your shoulders, and widens the space between your vertebrae. In addition, it synchronizes breathing and movement.

If you can bend and stretch your spine consciously, you can check and correct your posture throughout the day.

Sit down on a chair, and distribute your weight evenly on both sit bones.

Position your feet hip width apart, and distribute your weight evenly on your feet. The outer edges of your feet are parallel to one another.

Align your knee joints above your ankles.

Pull your pelvis upright, stretch your spinal column, and extend the crown of your head upward.

Raise your sternum, and let your hands lie loosely on your thighs.

Align your chin parallel to the ground, and relax your face, lips, and tongue.

Breathe in and out deeply through your nose.

Exhale as you bend your spine vertebra by vertebra, starting at your tailbone and moving all the way up: lumbar, thoracic, and cervical spine. Bow your head at the end.

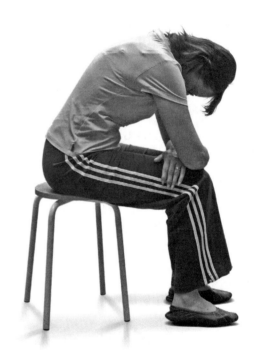

Inhale and stretch your spine vertebra by vertebra, starting at your tailbone and moving all the way up: lumbar, thoracic, and cervical spine. Lift your head at the end.

Repeat the bend and stretch exercise for six complete inhalations and exhalations.

Inhale, return to the seated posture, and relax.

Feel the effects of the exercise. Close your eyes if you like.

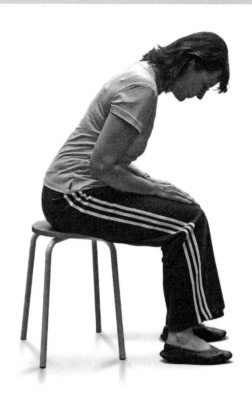

SQUAT

If you suffer from pain in your lower back, the squat is an easy and effective exercise. You can rest one hand on a chair or a handle bar for stabilization.

If you stay in squat for a long time, make sure that you rise slowly. Moving up suddenly might lead to a decrease in blood pressure and make you feel dizzy.

First come into mountain posture.

As you exhale, bend your knees, and come into squat.

Embrace your knees.

Focus on your back and let your shoulders and spine completely relax.

Maintain the position for at least three complete inhalations.

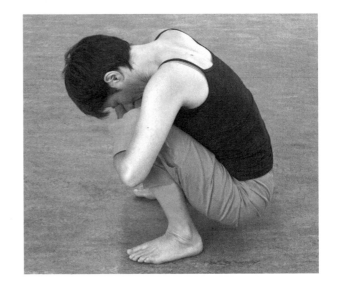

Variation

As you do the squat, stabilize your posture with your hands on the floor or holding a chair.

QUICK LOOK

Chapter 16 STRETCH AND RELAX YOUR BACK	
Mountain Posture	Immediately improves the feeling of strength, stretches the whole body, and helps to maintain balance, focus attention, and stand tall.
Turtle Posture	Relaxes the shoulders and enlarges the space between the vertebrae.
Tiger Breathing	Enhances your awareness of your spine, releases the tension in your shoulders, and enlarges the space between the vertebrae.
Squat	Immediately releases pain in the lower back and relaxes the shoulders.

17

Unburden Your Neck, Shoulders, and Arms

Often you are not aware that you are keeping your shoulders tight and pulled up for extensive periods of time until you feel pain or develop a headache.

Counter poor posture in your shoulders by regularly performing these exercises for the neck, shoulders, and arm muscles.

Keep in mind that after breast surgeries, it is vital to exercise hands, arms, and shoulders, especially after the removal of lymph nodes. The following exercises support the transport of tissue fluid back into the circulation (more postures in part II, chapters 6 and 7).

Practice with caution, making sure not to overdo the exercise.

ROTATIONS

Start with this exercise. Keeping your arms at shoulder level, gently move your shoulder joints and gain strength in your arm muscles.

Either kneel, stand, or sit with a stretched spine and your pelvis in an upright position.

Place your feet wider than hip width apart.

While breathing in through your nose, slowly raise your arms sideways to shoulder height.

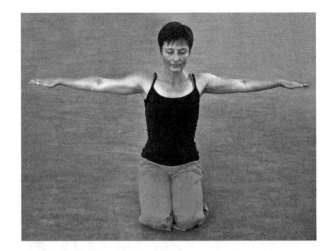

Make sure that you are raising your arms only, not your shoulders. If you are uncertain, briefly pull up your shoulders, and let them sink again.

As you exhale, rotate your stretched arms backward until your palms are facing back.

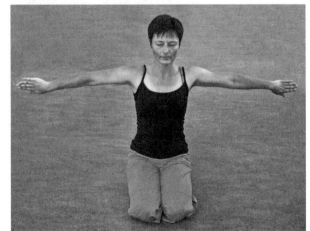

As you inhale, rotate your stretched arms forward until your palms are facing front.

Repeat this rotation for six complete breathing cycles.

Stop the movement. Inhale and stretch your arms again.

As you exhale, slowly lower your arms.

Return to the standing posture and feel the effects. Close your eyes if you like.

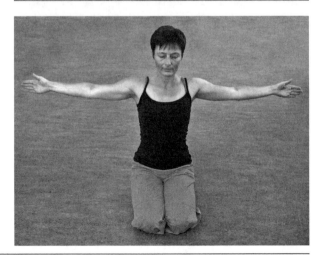

STRETCHES

This exercise, used to quickly relieve the feeling of heaviness in your arms, is a little more vigorous and should be done with caution.

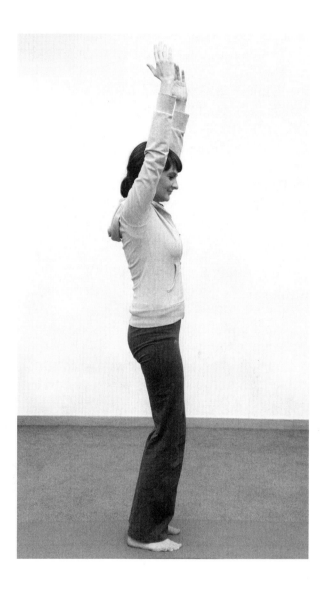

Come into the standing posture.

Place your feet hip width apart, and evenly distribute your weight on your feet.

Extend your knees (but do not hyperextend them), and rotate your thighs outward.

Tighten your pelvic muscles and stretch the vertebrae between your tailbone and the crown of your head.

Lower your chin toward your chest, and relax your shoulders and arms, as well as your face and tongue muscles.

Breathe in and out deeply through your nose.

As you inhale, lift your arms to the side raising your hands overhead and making sure not to lift your shoulders at the same time. Stretch your arms out as far as possible. Check if the stretch feels good, and, if not, reduce the stretch in one or both arms.

Open and close your hands (pumping).

Repeat the movement during six inhalations and exhalations.

As you exhale, lower your arms.

Feel the effect of the exercise. Close your eyes if you like.

BENDS

Arm bends train the muscles of the upper torso and support the transport of tissue fluid back into the circulation. You can intensify the effect if you make pumping movements with your hands (open and close your hands).

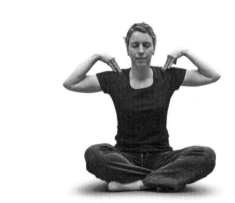

Either stand or sit with a stretched spine and your pelvis in an upright position.

Place your feet more than hip width apart.

While breathing in through your nose, slowly raise your arms sideways to shoulder height. Make sure that you are raising your arms only, not your shoulders. If you are uncertain, pull up your shoulders briefly, and let them sink again.

As you exhale, bend both arms.

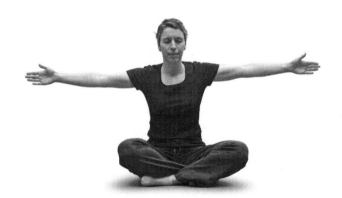

As you inhale, stretch out both arms.

Repeat the movements for six complete breathing cycles.

Stop the movement. Inhale and stretch your arms again.

As you exhale slowly lower your arms.

Return to the standing posture, and feel the effects. Close your eyes if you like.

Variation

Combine arm bends and hand exercises. As you exhale, bend both arms and close your hands, and as you inhale, stretch both arms and open your hands.

QUICK LOOK

	Chapter 17 UNBURDEN YOUR NECK, SHOULDERS, AND ARMS
Rotations	A gentle way to mobilize the shoulder joints and gain strength in arm muscles.
Stretches	A very efficient exercise to relieve the feeling of heaviness in the arms.
Bends	Trains the muscles and supports the transport of tissue fluid back into the circulation.

18

Concentrate
and
Focus

FOCUS NEAR AND FAR

Some women in our study reported that their vision seemed blurry after chemotherapy. Eye exercises train the eye muscles and relieve tension in the eyes.

You can do this posture discreetly during the day, whenever you have a few moments to yourself. If you have enough time to do the complete exercise, refer to part II chapter 5.

Sit on a chair with your spine stretched and your pelvis in an upright position, hands resting on your thighs.

Look at the tip of your nose, and breathe in and out.

Look at an object in near distance (for example, outstretched hand), and breathe in and out.

Look at an object that is close by, and breathe in and out.

Look at an object in the distance, and breathe in and out.

With the next inhalation, you no longer lock your eyes on an object. Instead, just look into the sky or ahead of you before breathing out again.

Repeat each step in reverse order until you are looking at your nose again.

Do the exercise six times.

Close your eyes, and feel the effect of the exercise.

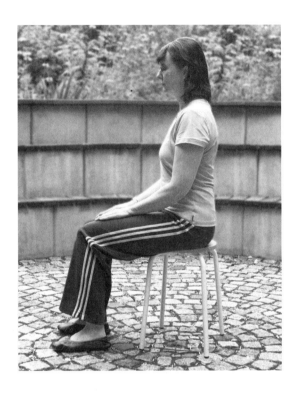

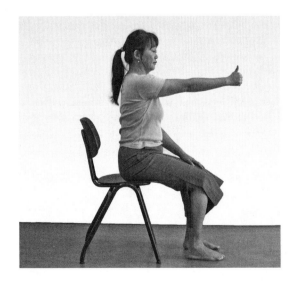

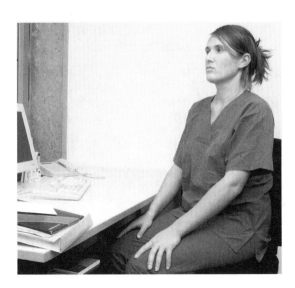

CUPPING AND BLINKING

After exercising the eye muscles, it is important to relax and moisten the eyes.

Keep your eyes closed, and rub your palms together. Completely cover your closed eyes with your warm palms, and let your fingertips rest on your hair line, relaxing your eyes as you feel the warmth of your palms transfer to your eyes.

Hold the posture as long as you can feel the warmth of your palms.

While keeping your eyes closed, take your hands off, and relax your arms in your lap.

Start blinking your eyes, quickly at first and then slowly.

Finally, open your eyes and keep them open, relax your whole body, and feel the effects.

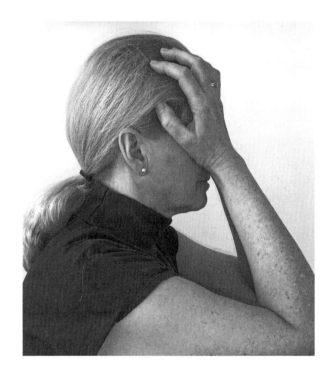

IMAGINATION

This posture, which you can perform anywhere, is a useful supplement to all arm, shoulder, and neck exercises because it energizes your arms without moving them and gives you the impression of a flowing motion in your vessels.

If you want to practice discreetly while on the bus or while you wait in a line, hold your hand bag on your lap or put your hands into your pockets. Make sure that your shoulders and arms are fully relaxed.

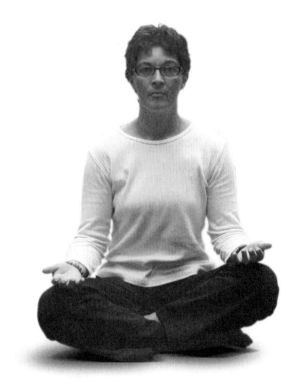

Sit upright on a chair. Stretch your spine, extend the crown of your head upward, align your chin parallel to the ground, and relax your shoulders and arms as well as your face and tongue muscles. Again, as you do this exercise, imagine energy moving up and down your arms.

Focus your attention on your left hand. Inhale through your nose, and move your attention up your left arm. Exhale through your nose, and move your attention to your right arm, then down to your hand.

Inhale through your nose, and move your attention up your right arm. Exhale through your nose, and move your attention down your left arm to your hand.

Repeat the exercise for six complete inhalations and exhalations.

ALTERNATE NOSTRIL BREATHING

Although this exercise has the best results for people suffering from asthma, we wanted to present it in this book—and regularly practiced it during our study—because alternate nostril breathing immediately widens the chest (bronchial tubes), helps you breathe evenly, relaxes the whole body, calms you, and increases awareness. On top of all that, it can be done anywhere.

Sit on a chair.

Bend the index finger, middle finger, and ring finger of one hand, and stretch out your thumb and little finger.

Place your thumb next to your right nostril and your little finger next to the left nostril. Either place your bent arm on the table, or hold it comfortably in front of your body in such a way that it is not pushing on your thorax and does not block your breathing.

To begin, first breathe out deeply through both nostrils.

Then close your right nostril with your thumb and slowly breathe in through your left nostril. Maintain the position, and feel your filled lungs.

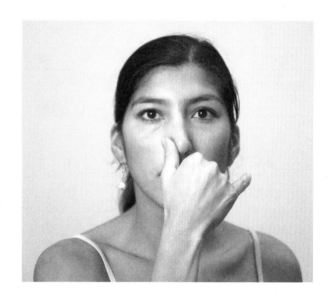

Close the left nostril with your little finger and slowly breathe out completely through the right nostril. Maintain the position, and feel your "empty" lungs.

Slowly breathe in again through the right nostril. Maintain the position, and feel your filled lungs. Close your right nostril with your thumb and slowly breathe out through the left nostril again. Maintain the position and feel your "empty" lungs.

Repeat the alternate nostril breathing for at least six complete breath cycles.

Finally, lower your hand and breathe in and out through both your nostrils. Feel the calming effects. Keep your eyes closed, if you like.

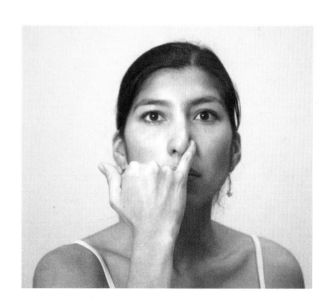

QUICK LOOK

Chapter 18 CONCENTRATE AND FOCUS	
Focus Near and Far	Counters blurry vision after chemotherapy, trains eye muscles, and relieves tension in the eyes.
Cupping and Blinking	Supports the relaxation of your eyes and facial muscles.
Imaginations	A supplement to all arm, shoulder, and neck exercises; energizes the arms and gives an impression of a flowing motion in the blood vessels.
Alternate Nostril Breathing	Widens the bronchial tubes, helps even breaths, relaxes the body, calms you, and supports awareness.

PART
IV

CONCENTRATION

AND

MEDITATION

YOGA MEDITATION

If you have already experienced meditative moments while practicing yoga postures and breathing exercises, you are well prepared for the next step: yoga meditation.

> *"It was helpful to be aware of the body during and after each yoga exercise. I felt my body, I was aware of my body, and I forgot about others and appointments and what to do next and tomorrow and next week."*

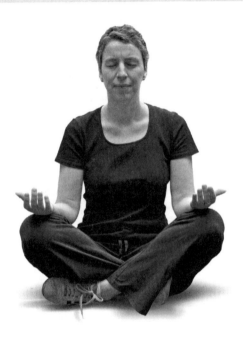

While practicing yoga postures, you are focused on your alignment and breath, which helps you relax by shifting the focus of your thinking, and by the end of a yoga class your mind is calm. Meditative exercises work similarly to get you into a quiet, relaxed mood. According to a number of studies, meditation has a positive, therapeutic effect because it alters brain waves, slows the heart beat, deepens breathing, and relaxes the muscles. Both traditional medicine and alternative therapy recommend meditation as a relaxation technique.

Many people think, incorrectly, that meditation is a passive activity. In fact, meditation requires much practice before you can fully benefit from the positive effects on the body and mind. Though the mention of meditation most often conjures images of Buddha sitting in the well-known lotus posture, this position is not usually the first position attempted because it requires the ability to remain in a sitting posture for a long period of time. For most people, it is easier to start with more active forms of meditation, such as walking, chanting, and singing.

Yoga offers a variety of methods for concentration and meditation, and there is no right way to move from working on your body to working on your meditative practice. As with the asanas and pranayama, meditation must be practiced regularly in order to become accustomed to how your body and mind respond to each posture. Here, we introduce two meditative yoga practices: pratyahara and dharana. These techniques train you to withdraw from the outside world and concentrate on yourself or on nothing at all.

WALKING MEDITATION

A lot of women in our study loved jogging, biking, and walking. Unfortunately, as with many types of exercises, they lacked the body awareness that is necessary for concentration and meditation. People often exercise without paying attention what they are doing; they listen to music instead of listening to their bodies. Many athletes end up ruining their hips and knees because their lack of care leads them to make mistakes, such as walking incorrectly, or wearing the wrong shoes.

One of the most straightforward methods of meditating involves the simple activity of walking. Walking meditation is beneficial when you feel restless and want to calm down. As you walk, concentrate on the various sensations you feel, from the pressure on the soles of your feet, to the warmth of your hands, to the movement of your knees and hips. Detach yourself from the outside world and concentrate on yourself. For best results, practice in a quiet space, such as a park or garden, an apartment, or a large room.

The easiest way to find out if walking is an effective form of meditation for you is to practice and experience it. If you already know you enjoy walking, find a private place, such as a short path around your yard. Start with five minutes, and slowly extend the time with each practice. As you walk, focus on every aspect of the activity, including how your joints feel, which parts of your body are relaxed and which are active. Note how long you can keep your attention focused, and celebrate your new ability.

YOGA NIDRA

Yoga nidra is a still form of meditation, during which your body and mind become completely relaxed. Lie down in shanti asana, and slowly become aware of your body part by part. You can develop your own path through your body or follow the words of a teacher, either in class or on a CD. Full instructions can be found in part II, chapter 9.

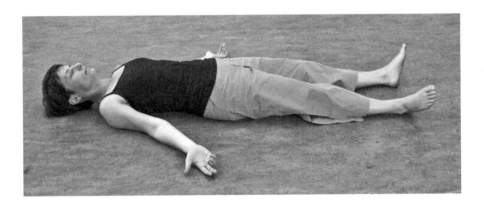

MANTRA MEDITATION

A mantra can be a syllable, a word, a line, a poem, or a song. You can choose a single word in English that means something important to you, such as silence, love, or confidence, or a word in Sanskrit, such as ananda (bliss), jaya (victory) or shanty (peace). Some people prefer to use the stanza of a poem, or even an entire song. Whatever you choose, recite it over and over, aloud or in your mind, with patience and resolution.

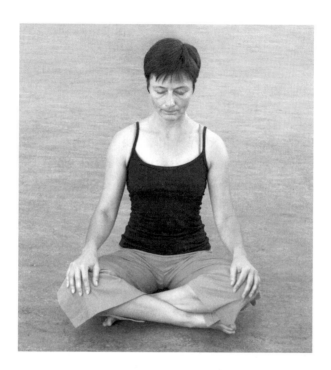

You may be familiar with the most famous yoga mantra, "OM." OM has many interpretations and, if you choose to use it, you may choose one that suits your needs and beliefs. Part of the appeal of OM is, undoubtedly, that it sounds good and can be recited or sung alone (either in your mind or aloud) and in groups (with everyone singing together or as a canon).

Another popular mantra, and one connected to breathing, is the sound "hamsa." In yoga, hamsa is called "the unpronounced mantra" because it is "continually produced by the body as a result of the breathing process. The syllable 'ham' is connected with inhalation, 'sa' with exhalation."[13] To perform this mantra, think or say "ham" while you are inhaling and "sa" while you are exhaling.

During our study, we ended each yoga lesson by chanting "aah" three times, "ooh" three times, and "mmm" three times. At first, the women were shy, chanting half-heartedly. The longer we practiced, the louder we got. Even new members in the group (there were new members each week) joined in, impressed by the energy they felt. Don't be afraid to try these things. They have no side effects and no definite meaning.

SOUND MEDITATION

Singing bowls have been used in individual and group yoga meditation for centuries. Made of metal or glass, they produce various tones—high, low, short, and long—when hit with a mallet. Sound meditation comes by concentrating for as long as possible on the sound produced. Become aware of how long you can focus your mind on the sound then refocus as the sound fades.

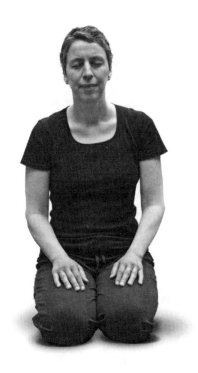

VISUAL MEDITATION

As the name implies, visual meditation requires focusing attention on a single object. In many representations of yoga, a candle is used, but any photo, written word, or object will do, and you can also just envision something in your mind. Concentrate on the object, real or imagined, for as long as possible. Become aware of how long you are able to maintain this attention.

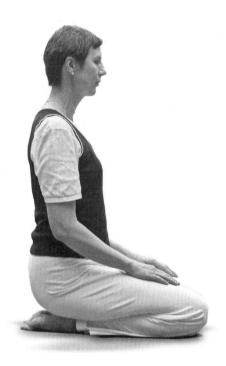

For women recovering from breast cancer or undergoing treatment, "white light," a healing light, has come to the fore as an effective visualization. The women in our study undergoing radiation told us that imagining white light going into the body made it easier for them to cope with the situation.

> *"Radiation is a torment. Day after day you have to go there, lie on that plank, alone in a room with a machine moving around you. You can't see anything, you can't feel anything, and you don't know what to think of it."*

"To imagine white light, healing light, floating through my body helped me find an explanation for what was going on and how it would help me. Fortunately, the time of radiation was very short and I could maintain the vision for the whole time."

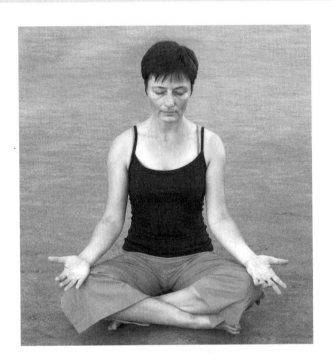

THINKING NOTHING AT ALL

As a patient you are exposed to an overwhelming amount of information—data, appointments, contacts, and conversations. Sometimes you may find it difficult to discriminate between what is important and what is not. The art of dharana allows you to give your thoughts a break, to stop listening, stop talking, and stop thinking. Through the practice of meditation, you can learn to experience a profound pause and to think nothing at all. Experiment with the methods we've described to determine which works best for you. As you gain experience, you will find it easy to slide into a time of no thought simply by meditating.

Be patient with yourself, enjoy each meditation, and always acknowledge your progress.

QUICK LOOK

Part IV CONCENTRATION AND MEDITATION	
Walking Meditation	A good meditative practice for beginners or for when you feel restless and want to calm down.
Yoga Nidra	Enhances the awareness of the body while in a comfortable posture, and improves sleep.
Mantra Meditation	A syllable, a word, a line, a poem, or a song in any language, recited again and again (aloud or in one's head).
Sound Meditation	Listening to a short ring or a long-lasting sound; for example, from singing bowls.
Visual Meditation	Focusing on an object or imagining white light streaming through the body.
Thinking Nothing at All	A demanding exercise designed to give your thoughts a break; to stop listening, stop talking, and stop thinking.

PART
V

USEFUL

INFORMATION

YOGA TRADITIONS

Most people think of yoga as a series of acrobatic positions, and headstands. The lotus posture could even be considered synonymous. However, this style of yoga, in which you attempt to achieve a consciousness of your own body, is relatively new. In the beginning, the center of yoga was spiritual-religious being. Early yoga was closely associated with Brahmanism, a religion previously connected with Hinduism, and was more about the transition of the body and complete spirituality, which was achieved by concentrating on meditation and prayer. Postures became a central theme only through their connection with the ability to maintain a meditative or prayer position motionlessly for long periods of time. Documents on yoga extend back to the Rig-Veda of the Keshin-Hymnus, dating to approximately 1200 BCE, and up to the Yoga Upanishad from 1600 CE.

Hatha Yoga, the most prominent form practiced today, takes the opposite approach. Rather than focusing on overcoming the body, the body and its well-being become the focus. The development of this style, in which yoga is considered physically uplifting, makes sense when the influence of old folklore traditions, which also had an influence on Indian religions, is taken into account. But while much is known about yoga through texts of the priests, historical sources on Hatha Yoga are sparse. The orientation toward the body appears to have been combined with the philosophic and religious roots of yoga and thus a visual language describing the body as a "temple of God" or "a place of pilgrimage and blessedness" developed. Besides the Patanjali Yoga Sutras, written roughly 2,000 years ago, the main texts of Hatha Yoga are the Yoga Upanishads (the oldest dated to 500 CE), the Gotaksha-Shataka (1200 CE), and the Hatha-Yoga-Pradipika (1400 CE).

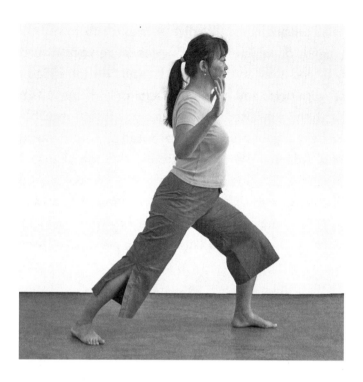

The historical developments of yoga can be traced back to well-known Sanskrit texts as well as to today's Indo-European languages. In his *Encyclopedia of Yoga*, Georg Feuerstein suggests the following as one possible lineage (p. 125):

- Archaic or Proto-Yoga (3000–1800 BCE), mentioned in the Vedic collections
- Preclassical Yoga (approximately 1500 BCE), documented in the early Upanishads
- Epic Yoga (500 BCE–200 CE), known from the Mahabharata—one of the two central Indian folklore epics (besides Ramayana) along with the well-known Bhagavad-Gita—as well as from the Upanishads of that time
- Classical Yoga (beginning of CE), in Patanjali's Yoga Sutras
- Postclassical Yoga (approximately 200 to 1900 CE), depicted in the Yoga Upanishads, Gotaksha-Shataka, and the Hatha-Yoga-Pradipika
- Modern Yoga, with various schools and ensuing literature

Yoga practice today can be quite diverse, and the form you choose to practice simply depends on which fits your needs. Since yoga is currently popular, you can easily attend a variety of yoga classes and decide which you like best.

Of course, yoga helps and becomes useful only through its practice. Start immediately with the exercises. The changes you feel in your body will establish its effectiveness in your mind and, motivated by your own experience, you can explore and understand the theoretical foundation of yoga. The literature on yoga is expansive, offering a wide variety of directions to deepen your knowledge. The Web pages of the best known Hatha Yoga traditions are listed below. As you read, continue to practice. The way yoga teachers live and pass on their traditions can be learned only through personal experience.

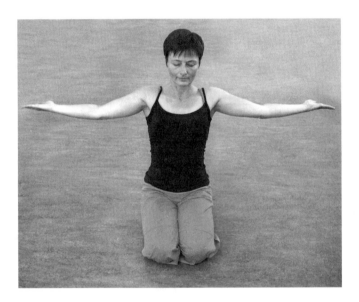

Note:

Easy accessibility to the place where you practice yoga is important because practicing regularly is paramount.

Good teachers are important because they must motivate and lead you.

A safe setting and individual support are important in adequately training you in handling your body, your thoughts, and your feelings.

Hatha Yoga Web Sites

Anusara: www.anusara.com
Ashtanga: www.ashtanga.com
Bikram: www.bikramyoga.com
Gitananda: www.gitanandayogasociety.com
Iyengar: www.iynaus.org
Jivamukti: www.jivamuktiyoga.com
Kundalini: www.3ho.org
Sivananda: www.sivananda.org
Triyoga: www.triyoga.com
Vini: www.viniyoga.com

Literature

1. Bower et al. *Cancer Control* 2005, 12(3), 165–171.
2. Brawley et al. *Control Clin Trials.* 2000, 21, 156–163.
3. Carlson et al. *Support Care Cancer* 2001, 9, 112–123.
4. Carlson et al. *Psychosom Med* 2003, 65, 571–581.
5. Carlson et al. *Psychoneuroendocrinology* 2004, 29, 448–474.
6. Carrico Yoga Journal's Yoga Basics: *The Essential Beginner's Guide to Yoga for a Lifetime of Health and Fitness*, 1997 (New York: Owl Book).
7. Carson et al. *J Pain Symptom Manage* 2007, 33, 331–341.
8. Casso et al. *Health Qual Life Outcomes* 2004, 2, 25.
9. Cohen et al. *Cancer* 2004, 100, 2253–2260.
10. Coulter: *Anatomy of Hatha Yoga. A Manual for Students, Teachers, and Practitioners*, 2001 (Honesdale, PA: Body and Breath).
11. Culos-Reed et al. *Psychooncology* 2006, 15, 891–897.
12. Danhauer et al. *Psychooncology* 2009, 18, 360–368.
13. Feuerstein: *The Shambhala Encyclopedia of Yoga* 2000 (Boston, London: Shambhala).
14. Fishman & Small: *Yoga and Mutiple Sclerosis. A Journey to Health and Healing* 2007 (Demos Medical Publishing).
15. Gross et al. *Psychophysiology* 2002, 39, 281–291.
16. Johnson et al. *Prev Med* 1998, 27, 56–64.
17. Kollak: *Yoga for Nurses* 2009 (New York: Springer Publishing Company).
18. Rao et al. *Eur J Cancer Care*, 2007.
19. Rosenbaum et al. *Support Care Cancer* 2004, 12, 293–301.
20. Snyder & Lindquist: *Complementary/Alternative Therapies in Nursing* 2006 (New York: Springer Publishing Company).
21. Telles et al. *Indian J Physiol Pharmacol* 1998, 42, 57–63.
22. Vempati et al. *Psychol Rep* 2002, 90, 487–494.

Index

Note: Boldface numbers indicate illustrations

Kollak, Ingrid.

Yoga and breast
cancer.

DATE			